AF316688

DEMYSTIFYING DIABETES

Unlock the secrets to Managing Diabetes, Control Blood Sugar, Improve Your Health, and Prevent Complications for a Better Life

Everyday Health Guide – Book -1

Dr. K. V. Sahasranam

Disclaimer

This book is based on authentic sources for its facts and statistics, with resources and references provided at the end. The opinions and conclusions presented are solely those of the author. While every effort has been made to keep the facts and details current, readers are encouraged to stay informed, as advancements in medicine occur at an exceptionally rapid pace. The names of the patients in the clinical scenarios presented have been changed to preserve their anonymity.

I dedicate this book

to my revered teachers of Medicine,

whose guidance instilled in me

the art and science of healing

and the wisdom to know when to intervene

and when to refrain.

My deepest gratitude and respect

are extended to each one of them.

ॐ सर्वे भवन्तु सुखिनः सर्वे सन्तु निरामयाः ।
सर्वे भद्राणि पश्यन्तु मा कश्चिद्दुःखभाग्भवेत् ।
ॐ शान्तिः शान्तिः शान्तिः ॥

Om Sarve Bhavantu Sukhinah, Sarve Santu Niraamayaah |
Sarve Bhadraanni Pashyantu, Maa Kashcid-Duhkha-Bhaag-Bhavet |
Om Shaantih Shaantih Shaantih ||

Om, May All be Happy, May All be Free from Illness.
May All See what is Auspicious, May no one Suffer.
Om Peace, Peace, Peace.

लोकाः समस्ताः सुखिनो भवन्तु

Loka samastha sukhino bhavanthu

May all beings everywhere be happy

A Humble Request to the Reader

Thank you for buying and reading this book. May I request your indulgence for one more favor.

I hope you enjoyed reading this book and derived benefit from the various topics discussed.

Kindly give your sincere and valuable review of this book in the Amazon site. Your rating and candid review will be a great inspiration and encouragement to me.

Please check out my other books given at the end of this book.

Check out my Website at **kvsauthor.com**

You can contact me at my email address

kvsauthor@gmail.com

TABLE OF CONTENTS

Chapter 1 - INTRODUCTION

Preamble

At the age of 50, just as the new century began, I received a diagnosis that would change my life: **Diabetes**. *Initially, it seemed manageable with small doses of oral medications, but over time, the challenges grew. My demanding career as a hospital physician, with its irregular hours and constant need to attend dinner meetings and conferences, made it difficult to maintain a strict diet and consistent exercise routine. As a result, my blood sugar levels fluctuated widely, and I found myself struggling to keep them under control.*

It was not until a warning from a trusted colleague, who was also managing my diabetes, that I realized the urgency of making a disciplined effort to take control of my health. With determination, I overhauled my lifestyle, adopting a strict dietary regimen and committing to regular exercise. The results were transformative. Now, nearly 25 years later, I am still on oral medications only, and my blood sugar is stable. I enjoy life without the fear of complications. I even indulge in sweets occasionally, knowing that I have the tools to manage my condition effectively.

This personal journey, marked by challenges and triumphs, inspired me to write this book. I wanted to share my experiences and the knowledge I have gained along the way with others who are navigating the complexities of diabetes. Whether you are newly diagnosed or have been living with the condition for years, this book aims to provide practical insights and empower you to take control of your health, just as I did.

Imagine waking up one morning and discovering that your body no longer processes sugar the way it used to. The foods you once enjoyed without a second thought are now potential threats to your well-being. Every meal becomes a careful calculation, every step a critical part of a new routine. This is the reality for millions of people living with diabetes—a condition that does not just affect your health but reshapes your entire life. But what if understanding this disease better could empower you to take control, make informed choices, and live a full, vibrant life despite diabetes? This book is your guide to doing just that. Whether you are newly diagnosed or supporting a loved one, "Demystifying Diabetes" will arm you with the knowledge and tools you need to navigate this journey with confidence. Let us embark on this path together, transforming challenges into opportunities for a healthier, happier future.

*   *   *   *   *

Diabetes mellitus is a chronic lifestyle disease characterized by an increase in blood levels of glucose. Glucose is the basic molecule in the body necessary for providing energy for the various bodily functions. When glucose is broken down to its components, energy is released which provides the impetus for all bodily functions. The brain is an organ which needs glucose to function efficiently, but it has no facility to store glucose. Hence a constant supply of glucose is needed by the brain even when the person is not feeding. So there is a need for maintaining a uniform supply of glucose in the blood always. This is facilitated by various mechanisms in the body.

There are two types of Diabetes described. One is called *Diabetes mellitus*. [*Diabetes* = siphon, *mellitus* = sweet]. The other is called *Diabetes insipidus* [*insipidus* = tasteless]. As the name suggests, the former is characterized by excretion of sweet urine and the latter by absence of sweetness in urine. Diabetes insipidus is due to a disease of the pituitary gland located within the brain and will not be discussed in this book.

'*Diabetes mellitus*', which will be hereafter referred to as 'diabetes' in this book is characterized by the excretion of glucose in urine. There are two types of diabetes – Type 1 Diabetes mellitus and Type 2 Diabetes mellitus abbreviated into **T1DM** and **T2DM** respectively. There are other rarer types of diabetes called *Maturity onset Diabetes in Adults* [**MODY**] and *Latent Autoimmune Diabetes in Adults* [**LADA**].

Some Important Technical Terms

Before proceeding further, let us briefly get acquainted with some terms used in this book which are derived from medical terminology.

Metabolism refers to the physical and chemical reactions in the body that change food into energy and those that use energy. They are the sum total of all chemical changes that take place in a cell or an organism. These changes generate energy and produce many other chemical substances that the cells and organisms need to grow, reproduce, and stay healthy. Metabolism also helps get rid of toxic substances from the body.

Homeostasis refers to any automatic process that a living being uses to keep its body steady on the inside while continuing to adjust to conditions outside of the body, or in its environment. The body makes these changes constantly to work and survive. A state of balance among all the body systems is needed for the body to survive and function correctly. Homeostasis is the ability to maintain a relatively stable internal state that persists despite changes in the world outside. For example, whether the surrounding temperature rises or falls, the human body remarkably maintains its internal temperature at a steady 37 degrees Celsius (98.6 degrees Fahrenheit). Similarly, the blood's pH is tightly regulated within the range of 7.35 to 7.45, ensuring the stability necessary for vital biochemical processes to occur seamlessly.

Oxidation is a chemical reaction that takes place when a substance reacts with oxygen or another oxidizing substance. It is a biological process that occurs in living cells when electrons are transferred from one compound to another. Oxidation is the loss of electrons during a reaction by a molecule, atom or ion. Examples of oxidation are rust and the brown color on a cut apple.

When we eat food, glucose is broken down in the presence of oxygen, leading to the production of energy, water, and carbon dioxide. The oxygen molecules act as the oxidizing agent, taking electrons from glucose. This oxidation process releases energy that the body uses to perform various functions. The liver uses oxidation to neutralize toxins in the body. For example, when alcohol is consumed, the liver oxidizes alcohol into acetaldehyde and then further breaks it down into acetic acid, which is less harmful and can be eliminated from the body. This process helps to detoxify the blood and prevent harmful substances from accumulating. This shows how oxidation maintains the body's energy levels and ensuring the removal of toxins.

Oxygen Free Radicals, also known as *Reactive Oxygen Species* (ROS) or *Free Radicals,* are unstable molecules that contain oxygen and one or more unpaired electrons. These unpaired electrons make the molecules more reactive, causing them to easily react with other molecules in a cell. It is a type of unstable molecule that contains oxygen and that easily reacts with other molecules in a cell. A buildup of oxygen radicals in cells may cause damage to the DNA, RNA, and proteins, and may cause cell death. Hence they are molecules detrimental to the body.

Autoimmunity is a condition where the body's immune system mistakes its own healthy tissues as 'foreign' and attacks them. A healthy immune system defends the body against attack by external agents like bacteria or viruses. The immune system produces proteins called **Antibodies** which attack external agents like bacteria, viruses and toxins and destroy them. An antibody produced against one's own tissues is called an **Autoantibody.**

Antioxidant is a substance that protects cells from the damage caused by Oxygen Free Radicals or Oxidants. The substances that act against these free radicals are called *Antioxidants.* Antioxidants thus minimize the damage caused by oxidants. Antioxidants protect us against cardiovascular disease, cancer and cataract and they slow down the effect of ageing. Examples of the most important antioxidants are vitamin C, vitamin E and beta-carotene. Plant foods abound in antioxidants. Fruits and vegetables are rich in them. Nuts, some types of meat, poultry and fish also contain antioxidants. Coffee contains powerful antioxidants. The body also produces certain antioxidants like *Glutathione* and *Alpha lipoic acid.*

Body Mass Index (BMI) is a measure of body fat based on the height and weight of a person. It is applicable for adults. BMI is calculated by dividing the weight (in kilograms) by the square of the height (in meters). It can also be calculated by dividing the weight in pounds by the square of the height in inches multiplied by a conversion faction of 703.

$$\text{BMI} = \underline{\text{Weight (in Kg)}} \div$$

$$\text{Height (in meters)}^2$$

$$\text{BMI} = \left[\frac{\underline{\text{Weight (in pounds)}} \div}{(\text{Height (in inches)})^2} \right] \times \mathbf{703}$$

A general rule of thumb to determine your ideal weight is as follows: subtract 100 from your height in centimeters. The result is your ideal weight. For instance, if your height is 160 centimeters (5'4"), your ideal weight would be 160 minus 100, which equals 60 kilograms.

Prevalence And Demographics

Prevalence refers to the number of people currently diagnosed with a disease in a community or a country.

Incidence refers to the number of new cases being diagnosed over a period, usually one year.

Both measures are needed to help assess the risk and burden of diseases on a community. It is found that the incidence of diabetes (the number of new cases occurring per year) has been increasing globally since 1990. One reason attributed to this is the increase in childhood obesity.

According to the estimates from the Centers for Disease Control and Prevention, in 2015, about 12.2% of U.S. adults were living with diabetes, including one in four adults aged 65 and older. This was the prevalence in 2015. The data shows a concerning trend in the prevalence of diabetes among US adults. Between 2002 and 2012, the incidence of type 1 diabetes in U.S. youths rose by 1.4%, while type 2 diabetes saw a more significant increase of 7.1%. Among those aged 10–19 years, the incidence of type 2 diabetes increased from 9.0 per 100,000 in 2002–2003 to 13.8 per 100,000 in 2014–2015. During the same period, the incidence of type 1 diabetes among all youths increased from 19.5 per 100,000 to 22.3 per 100,000. This data highlights the growing impact of diabetes on both adults and young people in the U.S. According the Centers for Disease Control and Prevention (CDC), in 2021, diabetes affected approximately 38.1 million Americans, accounting for 14.7% of the population. The prevalence of diagnosed diabetes varies across different racial and ethnic groups:

<u>American Indians/Alaskan Natives</u>: 13.6% of adults in this group have been diagnosed with diabetes, reflecting the highest prevalence among all racial and ethnic backgrounds.

<u>Non-Hispanic Black Adults</u>: 12.1% of this population is living with diabetes, highlighting a significant health concern within this community.

<u>Hispanic Adults</u>: With 11.7% affected, diabetes is also highly prevalent in the Hispanic population, underscoring the need for targeted health interventions.

<u>Asian American Adults:</u> 9.1% of adults in this group have been diagnosed with diabetes, showing a substantial impact within the Asian American community.

<u>Non-Hispanic White Adults</u>: 6.9% of this population has diabetes, marking the lowest prevalence among the racial and ethnic groups listed.

This data emphasizes the widespread impact of diabetes across the U.S., with certain communities facing a particularly high burden. Understanding these disparities is crucial for developing effective prevention and management strategies.

As per the Indian Council of Medical Research (ICMR) the total number of patients with diabetes in India in 2023 was 101 million. The prevalence of diabetes in India in 2023 has been reported to be 11.3%. China has around 141 million diabetics (2024), a prevalence of 11.2% as reported in 2020.

All this goes to prove that there is tremendous variability in the incidence and prevalence of diabetes depending on the ethnicity and geographic distribution of the population.

What is the importance of understanding diabetes?

Diabetes significantly affects both health and everyday life. In the short term, it can lead to serious health issues like *Diabetic Ketoacidosis*, which is a severe complication caused by high blood sugar levels, and a *Hyperglycemic Hyperosmolar State*, another dangerous state of very high blood sugar. Over time, diabetes can cause long-term health problems such as heart disease, nerve damage, vision problems, and kidney disease. Managing diabetes daily can be a heavy burden, requiring constant monitoring and lifestyle adjustments.

The economic impact of diabetes is also substantial. Managing diabetes can be expensive, involving costs for medications, blood sugar monitoring supplies, and frequent medical visits. This is particularly so in countries like India where the insurance coverage is insufficient. Beyond these direct costs, there are indirect costs to consider, such as lost productivity at work and potential disability due to diabetes-related complications.

From a public health perspective, diabetes is a major concern. Public health policies and programs often focus on reducing the prevalence and impact of diabetes. Health organizations work tirelessly to raise awareness, promote healthy lifestyles, and improve access to care to lessen the burden of diabetes on individuals and communities.

How To Use This Book

This book aims to educate readers about diabetes in an engaging and easy-to-understand manner. I have offered practical tips for managing diabetes effectively and to clear up common misconceptions by providing accurate, evidence-based information. The content is designed for people diagnosed with diabetes, their family members and caregivers, and anyone interested in learning more about the condition.

The book discusses the metabolism of glucose in some detail, but this may not be needed for many readers. I have included it only for completeness. To help with understanding, many of the technical and medical terms used in the book, they are explained in brackets in italics in the text itself. Therefore, a separate glossary is not included at the end.

The history of diabetes and the discoveries related to it make for fascinating reading. For those who wish to explore the history of diabetes, I have included a short chapter on this topic at the beginning of the book. The story of how diabetes has been understood and treated over the centuries is truly captivating. In this chapter, readers will learn about the early observations and descriptions of diabetes from ancient civilizations. The chapter highlights significant milestones in diabetes research, including the discovery of insulin and the development of modern treatments.

Readers might observe that some details about the disease are mentioned more than once throughout different chapters of this book. This repetition is deliberate. It ensures that even if someone chooses to focus on just one or two chapters, they still get the complete information and context necessary for a full understanding. Each chapter is designed to function independently, allowing readers to engage with any section they find relevant without needing to follow the book in its entirety or in a particular order. By doing this, I aim to make the content more flexible and accessible for those who may not read the book from start to finish. Reiterating key points also helps reinforce important information for those who may be browsing specific topics of interest. Thus, whether readers decide to explore just a single chapter or multiple sections, they will still gain valuable insights and not miss out on the essential aspects of the disease that are covered in this book. This approach allows for a more versatile reading experience, catering to both casual and thorough readers alike. At the start of each chapter, you will find a brief introductory paragraph that highlights the key points covered. This overview gives the reader a quick snapshot of what to expect, helping the reader get a clear sense of the chapter's content and main themes before diving into the details.

In various chapters of this book, you will find patient scenarios that illustrate real-life experiences with diabetes. These stories are based on true cases from the author's medical practice, providing valuable insights into how diabetes affects individuals in different ways. To protect the privacy of these patients, their names have been changed. These scenarios are included to help you understand the challenges and successes in managing diabetes, offering practical examples that you can relate to in your own journey or that of someone you care for. By reading these, you will gain a deeper appreciation for the complexities of living with diabetes and the importance of proper management and support.

An ***Appendix*** is included at the end, which provides _Conversion Tables_ for some commonly mentioned measurements in the text. For example, those in the United States may be more familiar with measurements like pounds, inches, and ounces, while readers in countries like India and

UK are more accustomed to metric units like grams, kilograms, liters, and meters. These tables will help make the information accessible to everyone, regardless of the measurement system they use.

Additionally, a list of references and recommended reading is appended at the end of the book. This list is for readers who want to seek more detailed academic information regarding diabetes.

Towards the end of the book, the reader will find a dedicated chapter on diet and nutrition. This, however, is far from complete. While it is impossible to cover every recipe and meal plan for all tastes, I have included a selection of recipes from the United States and India, featuring both vegetarian and non-vegetarian options. This variety aims to offer something to everyone. For more details on diet for diabetes, readers are referred to books specifically on 'Diets in Diabetes' by nutritionists and dietitians. This is because dietary needs can vary greatly from region to region and country to country. By referring to specialized books, readers can find information that is most relevant to their own dietary habits, tastes and preferences. Towards the end of the book, there is a chapter dedicated to *Resources and Support Groups*. This chapter also highlights useful apps that can benefit people with diabetes. It provides valuable information on where to find help and tools that can make managing diabetes easier and benefit the patients.

Overall, I hope this book serves as a valuable resource for those looking to understand and manage diabetes effectively. My goal is to empower readers with the knowledge and tools they need to live healthier, more informed lives.

Chapter 2 - HISTORY OF DIABETES

Diabetes is a disease with a long history, having been described by many ancient civilizations including the Egyptians, Indians, and others. The Ebers papyrus, dating back to 1550 BC, provides one of the earliest references to diabetes. In ancient India, during the 5th and 6th centuries BC, Ayurvedic physicians – Susrutha and Charaka, observed that the urine of some patients had a sweet taste. They called this condition '*Madhumeha*', which translates to "honey urine." Later physicians gave the name '*Prameha*' to the disease, a name still in use in India today.

Similarly, traditional Chinese medicine practitioners recognized the symptoms of diabetes and referred to it as '*Xiao ke*', meaning "*wasting thirst.*" Physicians from the medieval Islamic world also documented their observations and understanding of the disease in their medical writings. It was Demetrius of Apamea in the first century BC who is credited with naming the condition "*diabetes*", which means '*siphon*' or '*pass through*'. Roman writers like Celsus [30 BC – 50 AD] also have provided an early description of diabetes.

Significant advancements in the understanding of diabetes continued over the centuries. In 1794, a German physician named Johann Peter Frank made a crucial distinction between two types of diabetes: Diabetes mellitus and Diabetes insipidus. This differentiation helped in understanding that the conditions, while similar in some symptoms, had different underlying causes. Further progress was made in 1889 when Joseph von Mering and Oskar Minkowski discovered the role of the pancreas in causing diabetes. This discovery was pivotal in advancing the medical community's understanding of the disease and paved the way for future research and treatment options.

In 1869, a German pathologist and physiologist named Paul Langerhans made a significant discovery within the pancreas. He identified clusters of cells that were different from the cells responsible for secreting pancreatic juice. In recognition of his contribution, these cell clusters were named the *"Islets of Langerhans."*

As scientific understanding progressed towards the end of the 19th century and the beginning of the 20th century, researchers began to theorize that these islets produced a specific substance. They named this substance *"Insulin"* and believed it played a crucial role in the metabolism of carbohydrates in the body.

A breakthrough occurred when Nicolae Constantin Paulescu, a Romanian physician, conducted an experiment involving a diabetic dog. He injected an extract made from the pancreas into a diabetic dog and observed that its blood sugar levels returned to normal. This finding was revolutionary. Paulescu identified the extract as insulin confirming its vital role in managing blood sugar levels. This discovery was a crucial moment in diabetes research, opening new avenues for treatment and understanding of the disease.

The history of understanding diabetes pathology is equally fascinating. In 1788, Thomas Cawley conducted an autopsy on a diabetic patient and observed damage to the pancreas. This led him to hypothesize that the disease originated in the pancreas. Building on this idea, Joseph von Mering and Oskar Minkowski performed an experiment in 1889 where they removed the pancreas from a dog, which subsequently developed diabetes. This experiment further solidified the link between the pancreas and diabetes.

In 1893, Edouard Hedon carried out another significant experiment. He removed the pancreas from a dog, just as von Mering and Minkowski had done, but then he implanted a small section of the pancreas under the dog's skin. Remarkably, the dog did not develop diabetes, suggesting that even a small part of the pancreas could prevent the onset of the disease. These series of discoveries and experiments paved the way for a deeper understanding of diabetes and the critical role of the pancreas in its development. The treatment of diabetes also bears an interesting history.

In 1921, a groundbreaking discovery was made at the University of Toronto by a team of researchers including Frederick Banting, John Macleod, Charles Best, and James Collip. They successfully discovered and purified insulin, making it suitable for clinical use in treating diabetes. In a remarkable gesture of generosity and commitment to public health, they sold the patent for insulin to the University of Toronto for just one dollar. This symbolic act ensured that the treatment would remain accessible and affordable for everyone who needed it.

The history of diabetes treatment is just as intriguing as the discovery of the disease itself. Before the mid-1800s, the methods used to treat diabetes were quite primitive and varied. Physicians often relied on a mixture of strange ingredients, including bloodletting and opium. Additionally, they would give patients excessive amounts of food to make up for the sugar lost in their urine. These treatments were largely ineffective and sometimes even harmful.

An important turning point came when Appollinaire Bouchardat made a noteworthy observation during the Franco-Prussian War in Paris in 1870. Bouchardat noticed that rationing and the resulting starvation led to a significant reduction in the amount of sugar excreted in the urine of diabetic patients. This improvement in the condition of patients highlighted the potential benefits of a diet low in sugar and carbohydrates. His observations laid the groundwork for dietary modifications as a treatment for diabetes.

Building on these findings, F.M. Allen introduced what became known as the *"Starvation diet."* This diet was designed to restrict caloric intake severely, aiming to reduce the burden on the body's metabolism and control blood sugar levels more effectively. Although extreme by today's standards, this approach marked a significant shift towards dietary management in treating diabetes and demonstrated the impact of food intake on the disease. This historical progression underscores the evolution of diabetes treatment from unscientific remedies to more systematic and research-based approaches.

The structure of insulin was delineated in 1955 by Fred Sanger. The first pancreas transplant was performed by William Kelly, Richard Lillehei and others at the University of Minnesota in 1972.

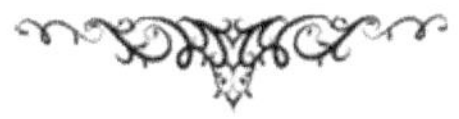

Chapter 3 - GLUCOSE METABOLISM

In this chapter, we will explore how the body processes glucose, a vital source of energy. We will discuss how glucose is absorbed from the food we eat, how it enters our bloodstream, and how insulin helps move it into our cells. We will learn about the role of the pancreas in producing insulin and how this hormone regulates blood sugar levels. We will also cover what happens when this process goes awry, as in diabetes, leading to either high or low blood sugar levels. Understanding glucose metabolism is essential for managing diabetes effectively. This knowledge will empower one to make informed decisions about diet, lifestyle, and treatment options to maintain optimal blood sugar levels and overall health.

Normal Glucose Metabolism

<u>Overview of Glucose Metabolism</u>:   Glucose is a of type sugar that serves as the main energy source for the body. It is essential for providing energy to all our cells so that they can function properly. It is derived from the food we eat,

especially from foods rich in carbohydrates like bread, pasta, rice, and fruits. When we eat these foods, our body breaks them down into glucose through the process of digestion in the gut.

<u>Absorption and Utilization:</u>   On eating carbohydrate-rich foods, our digestive system with the aid of the digestive juices in the stomach and the intestines, starts breaking them down into smaller sugars. A major part of this is glucose. After carbohydrates are broken down in the small intestine, the glucose thus formed is absorbed into the bloodstream and is carried to all parts of the body.

The body's cells need glucose for energy. To get the glucose inside the cells, it must pass through the cell membrane. The cell membrane is a thin biological membrane that protects the inside of the cell from its external environment. This process of glucose entry into the cell is helped by special proteins called *Glucose Transporters*. These proteins act like doors, allowing glucose to enter the cells from the blood. Once inside the cells, glucose is used to produce energy that powers all the activities of the body.

Let us get acquainted with some terms used in the metabolism of glucose in the body and learn the steps in glucose metabolism in a simple manner.

<u>Glycolysis</u> is the process in which glucose is broken down step by step into smaller molecules. This breakdown happens in a series of biochemical reactions that occur inside the cells. The main role of glycolysis is to produce energy. During glycolysis, glucose is converted into a chemical named Pyruvate in a series of biochemical reactions, and during this process energy is released which the cells utilize for their various functions.

<u>Glycogenesis</u> is another process where the body takes the surplus glucose that is not immediately needed for energy and converts it into a chemical named *Glycogen*. The glycogen

thus formed is stored in the liver and muscles. This stored glycogen can be used later when the body needs more energy, as between meals or during physical activity by breaking it back into glucose.

Glycogenolysis is another chemical reaction that is the opposite of glycogenesis. It is the process where the stored glycogen in the liver and muscles is broken down back into glucose. This happens when the body needs more glucose, such as during fasting or vigorous exercise. The glucose thus released from glycogen can be used by the cells for energy.

Gluconeogenesis is the process where the body produces glucose from non-carbohydrate sources like amino acids which are derived from proteins or lactate obtained from muscle activity. This process is crucial when there is not enough glucose available from food or glycogen stores. The liver and kidneys play important roles in this process. They perform gluconeogenesis to ensure a steady supply of glucose in the body, especially during times of fasting or when the body needs extra energy. It is to be noted that *gluconeogenesis* is different from *glycogenesis*.

Maintaining Blood Glucose Levels: The body has a mechanism to keep the blood level of glucose within a specific range, which is between 70 and 110 mg/dL. This has been named *Homeostasis*, which we have seen already in chapter 1. This range is important because it ensures that there is enough glucose available always for the body's needs without having too much or too little. This regulation involves various feedback mechanisms that function to adjust the blood levels of glucose. For example, when blood glucose levels increase after eating, the body responds by releasing insulin to help lower the glucose levels. When blood glucose levels drop, as occurs between meals or during exercise or fasting, other hormones help to increase glucose levels by releasing stored glucose from the glycogen in the liver.

Insulin: Insulin is a hormone produced and released by the beta cells of the pancreas. When one takes food and the blood sugar rises, these beta cells sense the increase and release insulin into the bloodstream. Insulin thus released acts by facilitating the entry of glucose through the cell membrane. It acts like a key that unlocks the doors to the cells, allowing glucose to enter where it can be used for energy.

In addition to helping with glucose uptake, insulin also has other important actions.

- It helps the conversion of glucose into glycogen, which is then stored in the liver and muscles.
- Insulin also aids in the production and storage of fats through a process called *Lipogenesis.*
- Insulin also aids in synthesizing proteins in the body.
- Insulin blocks the production of new glucose in the liver, (*gluconeogenesis*).
- It blocks the breakdown of glycogen back into glucose, (*glycogenolysis*).

Thus, the level of glucose is always kept within the physiological range by the actions of insulin.

Other hormones that affect blood glucose levels.

Glucagon: Glucagon is another hormone produced by the Alpha cells of the pancreas. These cells release glucagon into the bloodstream when blood sugar levels are low, such as between meals, during exercise or while fasting. The main action of glucagon is to raise blood glucose levels. It does so by signaling the liver to break down stored glycogen into glucose (*glycogenolysis*). Additionally, glucagon also induces the liver to produce new glucose from non-carbohydrate sources (*gluconeogenesis*). Thus, insulin and glucagon work together to maintain the balance of glucose in the blood. When blood glucose is high, insulin lowers it, and when it is low, glucagon raises it. This remarkable teamwork ensures that the body always has a steady supply of glucose for energy.

Cortisol: Cortisol is a hormone released by the adrenal glands, especially during times of stress. It is also called the *"Stress hormone"*. Its main role is to help the body respond to stress, but it also has important effects on blood glucose levels. When cortisol levels increase in blood, it promotes gluconeogenesis thereby increasing blood levels of glucose. Cortisol also makes the body less sensitive to insulin, which again leads to higher blood sugar levels. This is the body's mechanism to ensure enough energy to handle stressful situations. Note that the action of cortisol and insulin are antagonistic to each other.

Epinephrine (Adrenaline):   Epinephrine, also known as adrenaline, is a hormone released by the adrenal glands during stress or the *'fight or flight'* response. This hormone prepares the body to respond quickly to danger. One of the ways epinephrine does this is by raising blood glucose levels thus ensuring enough energy for the body to face any danger or crisis. It also signals the liver to break down glycogen into glucose, providing a quick source of energy. Epinephrine also reduces the amount of insulin released by the pancreas, which helps keep blood glucose levels high. All these ensure that muscles and other tissues have enough energy to respond to a threat.

Growth Hormone: Growth hormone is produced by the pituitary gland. It plays an important role in regulating growth and metabolism in the body. It also impacts the blood glucose levels. This hormone acts by making the cells less sensitive to insulin, which can lead to higher blood glucose levels. Growth hormones also stimulate gluconeogenesis, thus increasing blood glucose levels. These actions provide energy needed during periods of growth and development.

Other Hormones: There are several other hormones that also play a role in glucose metabolism. *Incretins* are a group of hormones released from the intestines in response to eating. They help to promote insulin secretion to ensure proper control of blood glucose levels after a meal. *Adipokines* are hormones produced by fat tissue that influence how the body handles glucose. For example, one such hormone named *Leptin* helps regulate appetite and energy balance, while another named *Adiponectin* enhances insulin sensitivity, helping to lower blood glucose levels. These hormones contribute to the overall regulation of glucose metabolism and help maintain stable blood sugar levels.

Let us see how diabetes can have an impact on glucose metabolism.

Type 1 Diabetes

Type 1 diabetes (T1DM) occurs when the body's immune system mistakenly attacks and destroys the beta cells in the pancreas that produce insulin. Without insulin, the body cannot properly regulate blood glucose levels. Insulin is essential for helping glucose enter the cells where it can be used for energy. In the absence of insulin, glucose levels rise in the bloodstream leading to high blood sugar levels. People with T1DM thus must rely on external sources of insulin, often through injections or an insulin pump, to manage their blood glucose levels. They need to monitor their blood sugar levels regularly and adjust their insulin doses. to simulate the natural fluctuations of insulin in the body and maintain more stable glucose levels.

Type 2 Diabetes

Type 2 diabetes (T2DM) is characterized by the cells becoming less responsive to insulin due to *Insulin Resistance*. Even though the pancreas still produces insulin, it is not as effective at helping glucose to enter the cells. To overcome this insulin resistance, the pancreas begins to produce more and more insulin. Gradually, the pancreatic beta cells in people with T2DM may become exhausted from overworking and producing extra insulin. Eventually, they fail to produce enough insulin to keep blood sugar levels in check, leading to higher blood glucose levels. Insulin resistance affects the body's ability to take up glucose from the blood, convert glucose to glycogen for storage, and produce glucose through gluconeogenesis. These can lead to elevated blood sugar levels, which increase the risk of complications such as cardiovascular disease, nerve damage, and kidney problems.

Chronic Hyperglycemia

Chronic hyperglycemia refers to consistently high blood glucose levels over an extended period. This can cause damage to various organs and tissues throughout the body. High blood sugar levels lead to the formation of harmful molecules called *Advanced Glycation End products* (**AGEs**). AGEs can damage blood vessels and tissues, causing complications like damage to the retina of the eye (*Retinopathy*), the nerves (*Neuropathy*), and kidneys (*Nephropathy*). Hence, keeping the blood glucose levels within a normal range is crucial to prevent these complications.

Hypoglycemia

Hypoglycemia, which means low blood glucose levels occurs when the levels are too low. This can happen if a person with diabetes takes too much insulin, skips meals, or engages in intense physical activity. The symptoms of hypoglycemia include shakiness, sweating, confusion, irritability, and even loss of consciousness if left untreated. These symptoms should be recognized early and treated. To prevent hypoglycemia regular blood sugar monitoring, eating regular meals and snacks, adjusting insulin doses as needed, and carrying a fast-acting source of glucose, like candy or glucose tablets is needed. [See chapter 8 on *Complications of Diabetes*].

Metabolic Dysfunction

Diabetes affects lipid metabolism, leading to an abnormal balance of fats in the blood. This condition is called *Dyslipidemia*. This can increase the risk of heart disease and stroke. Diabetes can also alter protein metabolism, leading to muscle wasting and weakness. Hence, maintaining a balanced diet and regular physical activity is important for managing these metabolic changes and preserving muscle mass.

Diabetic Ketoacidosis (DKA)

Diabetic ketoacidosis is an acute serious complication that can occur in people with T1DM. It happens when the body starts breaking down fats for energy due to a lack of insulin, leading to the production of chemicals called *Ketones*, which are acidic. Insulin deficiency and increased fat breakdown (*lipolysis*) results in the levels of ketones to increase in blood. Symptoms like nausea, vomiting, abdominal pain, and even coma can occur if prompt treatment is not given. DKA requires immediate hospitalization and medical attention. It is treated with fluids, electrolytes, and insulin to lower blood glucose levels and block the production of ketones. [See chapter 8 on *Complications of Diabetes*].

Hyperosmolar Hyperglycemic State (HHS)

Hyperosmolar hyperglycemic state is also a severe complication that can occur in people with T2DM. It is characterized by extremely high blood glucose levels and severe dehydration. In HHS, the high blood glucose levels cause the blood to become thick and syrupy (*hyperosmolar*). As the body tries to excrete the excess glucose through urine, the person becomes dehydrated. The symptoms are extreme thirst, frequent urination, dry skin, and confusion. HHS is a medical emergency that requires immediate hospitalization with rehydration, insulin therapy, and careful monitoring to prevent complications and restore normal blood glucose levels. [See chapter 8 on *Complications of Diabetes*].

Poorly controlled blood glucose levels, whether too high (*hyperglycemia*) or too low (*hypoglycemia*), can lead to a range of complications affecting various parts of the body. Hence, it is crucial for people with diabetes to manage their blood sugar levels effectively to prevent these complications.

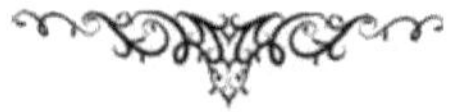

Chapter 4 - TYPES OF DIABETES

*Understanding the different types of diabetes is crucial for effective management and treatment. The main types of diabetes are Type 1, Type 2, and Gestational Diabetes, each with distinct characteristics and implications for health. Type 1 Diabetes (**T1DM**) is an autoimmune condition where the body's immune system attacks insulin-producing cells in the pancreas. This type usually develops in children and young adults, requiring lifelong insulin therapy. Type 2 Diabetes (**T2DM**) is the most common form, typically developing in adults. It is often linked to lifestyle factors such as obesity and inactivity, where the body becomes resistant to insulin or does not produce enough insulin. Gestational Diabetes (**GDM**) occurs during pregnancy and can pose risks to both mother and baby if not managed properly. There are also rarer forms of diabetes, such as Maturity-Onset Diabetes of the Young (**MODY**) and Latent Autoimmune Diabetes in Adults (**LADA**), which have unique diagnostic and treatment challenges. **Prediabetes** is a condition where the blood sugar is elevated more than normal but does not reach levels to be diagnosed as diabetes.*

The Pancreas: A Brief Description

Before getting into the details of the disease, let us briefly discuss the Pancreas which is a gland situated in the abdomen in our body and is a crucial organ involved in the disease. [**Fig 1**]

The pancreas is an important organ that plays a crucial role in digestion and blood sugar regulation. The pancreas is found in the upper part of the abdomen behind the stomach and close to the spine occupying the C-shaped curvature of the Duodenum, which is the first part of the small intestines. It is a leaf-shaped or tadpole shaped organ about 6 inches (15 cms) long. It has a mix of two types of tissues. There are tissue cells that secrete pancreatic juice which helps with digestion and those that regulate blood sugar. Thus, the pancreas helps both in digesting food and keeping the blood sugar levels balanced by producing important hormones.

The part of the pancreas that controls blood sugar contains small groups of cells called the *Islets of Langerhans*. These are tiny clusters of different types of cells scattered throughout the pancreas. There are three main types of cells in these islets:

1. **Alpha Cells**: They produce a hormone called *Glucagon*, which raises blood sugar levels.

2. **Beta Cells**: They produce *Insulin*, a hormone that lowers blood sugar levels. These cells are   crucial for managing diabetes.

3. **Delta Cell**: They produce *Somatostatin*, which helps regulate the other two hormones.

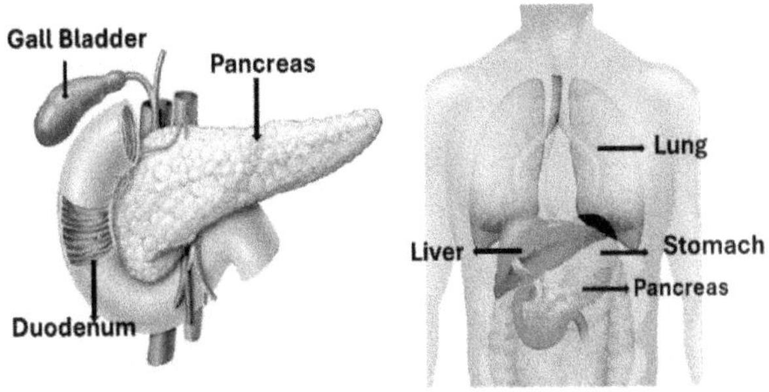

Figure 1 showing the pancreas and its location in the body.

Diabetes mellitus has been classified into different types based on the causation and onset of the disease. They are:

Type 1 Diabetes mellitus (T1DM) which is due to an Autoimmune process which destroys the insulin producing cells in the pancreas leading to insulin deficiency. This is the type seen often in children and may start in infancy also.

Type 2 Diabetes mellitus (T2DM) which is due to Insulin resistance which means that insulin is not able to function in the body even though it is produced in the pancreas. This is the type often seen in adults but not necessarily confined to them as has been seen in adolescents and children too.

Gestational Diabetes mellitus (GDM) which is the diabetes that appears for the first time in pregnancy and very often disappears after the child is born.

Prediabetes

Prediabetes is a condition where blood sugar levels are higher than normal but not yet high enough to be diagnosed as

T2DM. It is a warning sign that the individual is at risk of developing diabetes if healthy lifestyle changes are not made.

Prediabetes does not appear suddenly. A person may remain in the prediabetic stage for years together due to insulin resistance. All patients with prediabetes do not necessarily develop diabetes. Adopting a good lifestyle can prevent diabetes in many with prediabetes. But often many with prediabetes do not realize that they have the problem. Hence it is necessary to test the blood sugar of those over the age of 40. In some countries where diabetes is more common, the test is done earlier at the age of 35 or 30.

The following are the recommended indications to test for Prediabetes.

- Persons belonging to a high risk group – African Americans, Latinos, Asians, Native Americans.

- Persons with a high blood pressure.

- Persons in whom the good cholesterol fraction in blood (HDL) is low.

- Person in whom the Triglyceride levels in blood are high.

- Those with a family history of diabetes.

- If Gestational diabetes occurred or if the baby was overweight previously (more than 9 lbs.).

Twenty five percent of those with prediabetes develop the disease in 3-5 years. According to an American Diabetes

During a routine medical checkup, Sarah, a 26-year-old female lawyer, was found to have a fasting blood sugar level of 120 mg/dL. Her doctor diagnosed her with Prediabetes. The doctor explained that prediabetes is a warning sign and emphasized the importance of taking action to prevent the progression to type 2 diabetes. Sarah was advised to adopt several lifestyle changes to manage her condition effectively.

First, she needed to focus on her diet, incorporating more whole grains, vegetables, fruits, lean proteins, and reducing her intake of sugars and refined carbohydrates. Portion control and balanced meals were crucial. Second, Sarah was encouraged to increase her physical activity. Engaging in at least 150 minutes of moderate aerobic exercise, such as brisk walking or cycling, each week will be needed to help regulate her blood sugar levels.

Sarah took up playing tennis for an hour daily. Additionally, the doctor suggested regular monitoring of her blood sugar levels and follow-up appointments to track her progress. Sarah was also advised to maintain a healthy weight, as losing even a small amount of weight could significantly improve her blood sugar control. Sarah lost six pounds in three months. By making these changes, Sarah effectively managed her prediabetes and thereby reduced her risk of developing type 2 diabetes in the future.

Association (ADA) statement in 2013 up to 70% of people with prediabetes will eventually develop type 2 diabetes (T2DM)

Metabolic Syndrome

Metabolic syndrome (MS) is a health condition marked by a group of related problems, such as excessive belly fat, difficulty in using insulin properly, high blood pressure, and abnormal levels of fats in the blood. It is also known by other names such as *Insulin resistance syndrome, Dysmetabolic syndrome* and *Syndrome X*. It is a collection of conditions that raise the risk of diabetes, stroke, coronary heart disease, and other severe health issues. MS is seen in many persons with Prediabetes and often these patients develop frank diabetes later.

To diagnose someone with metabolic syndrome, doctors look for at least **three** of the following signs:

i. A waist size larger than 40 inches (100 cm) for men and 35 inches (90 cm) for women. For Asian individuals, the cutoff is 35 inches (90 cm) for men and 32 inches (80 cm) for women.
ii. High levels of triglycerides in the blood, specifically 150 mg/dL or higher.
iii. Low levels of high-density lipoprotein (HDL) cholesterol, which is less than 40 mg/dL for men and less than 50 mg/dL for women.
iv. High blood sugar levels when fasting, which is 100 mg/dL or greater.
v. High blood pressure, with readings of 130 mm Hg or higher for systolic pressure or 85 mm Hg or higher for diastolic pressure.

People with metabolic syndrome are twice as likely to develop heart diseases related to artery hardening and narrowing and five times as likely to develop diabetes compared to those without the condition.

The causes of metabolic syndrome are varied and include genetic factors as well as several lifestyle factors. Key contributors include being overweight, not getting enough exercise, and eating an unhealthy diet. The core issue in metabolic syndrome is the accumulation of fat tissue, particularly around the abdomen, which leads to the body's decreased ability to use insulin effectively.

Latent Autoimmune Diabetes in Adults (LADA)

This is seen in adults. It begins in adulthood and gradually worsens over time. It is due to an autoimmune process that damages the islet cells of the pancreas thereby reducing insulin secretion. It is a type 1 diabetes seen in adults but is often milder and slowly progressing.

Symptoms often start after the age of 30 and are the same as other types of diabetes. Unlike those with T2DM, patients with LADA are often not obese. The diagnosis is often made by detecting autoantibodies to islet beta cells in the blood of these patients. (See Chapter 7 on *Type 1 Diabetes mellitus*). A history of other autoimmune diseases may be present in the patient or other members of the family.

The management of these patients is often like that of T2DM. Initially they may not require insulin but later they become insulin dependent when the insulin producing beta cells of the pancreas are destroyed. Complications like ketosis are rare in this type of diabetes.

Maturity Onset Diabetes of the Young (MODY)

It is seen in non-obese children, adolescents and early adulthood and constitutes only a small proportion of patients with diabetes. Often it begins before the age of 25. In the US about 5% of diabetes cases belong to this category. It is genetically mediated caused by the mutation of a single gene. (*Monogenic Mutation*) and is due to ineffective insulin production. Often a family member has the disease. If a parent has the disease, there is a 50% chance that the children could inherit it. Genetic studies may be done to diagnose the condition and identify the specific gene responsible for the mutation. It is treated with oral medications or insulin injections.

We shall discuss each of the main types of diabetes separately in detail. LADA and MODY being uncommon have already been discussed here.

Rare Causes of Diabetes

Diabetes can also occur in certain other conditions as given below.

- Surgical removal of pancreas for cancer or multiple stones.
- *Hemochromatosis* is a condition where there is excess absorption of iron leading to heavy deposition of iron in the Pancreas, Liver, Heart, Joints and the Nervous system. It is a rare hereditary disease.
- Excess production of hormones that oppose insulin action e.g. Adrenal gland tumors producing excess corticosteroids or Pituitary gland tumors producing excess growth hormone.
- Medications causing diabetes are also seen occasionally. Hydrocortisone used in treatment of various diseases, certain medications like Hydrochlorothiazide used in the treatment of high blood pressure and some anti-inflammatory medications too may cause diabetes.

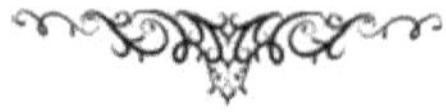

Chapter 5 - TYPE 2 DIABETES MELLITUS
Causes, Risk Factors, Symptoms & Diagnosis

Type 2 Diabetes (T2DM) is the most common form of diabetes, affecting millions of people worldwide. This chapter is dedicated to helping you understand the causes, risk factors, symptoms, and diagnosis of T2DM. It is essential to recognize that T2DM often develops gradually, making it crucial to be aware of the early signs and take action before complications arise. Understanding the risk factors, such as genetics, lifestyle choices, and other medical conditions, can empower you to make informed decisions about your health. This chapter will also guide you through the common symptoms of T2DM, such as increased thirst, frequent urination, and fatigue, so you can identify them early. Additionally, it will explain the various diagnostic tests used to confirm T2DM, providing you with a clear understanding of what to expect during the process.

We have seen that diabetes is a condition characterized by an increase in blood glucose to values more than normal.

This condition of high blood glucose is called *Hyperglycemia*. In Type 2 Diabetes (**T2DM**) there are mainly two problems. The pancreas produces less insulin than normal and the insulin that is produced is not able to function properly. The cells in the body's tissues are said to be 'resistant' to insulin, in other words, the person has Insulin Resistance. T2DM was previously called *Non-insulin dependent diabetes mellitus* (**NIDDM**).

Normally, insulin helps the circulating glucose to enter the cells to be utilized for production of energy. In insulin resistance, this entry of glucose into the cells is impaired and hence cells are not able to take up glucose to produce energy for its needs. The muscle cells cannot take up glucose for the muscles to contract properly and the brain cells cannot take up glucose properly to function normally. [See Chapter 3 on *Glucose Metabolism*].

CAUSES AND RISK FACTORS FOR T2DM

Some of the risk factors and causes of diabetes (both types 1 and 2) are discussed below in considerable detail. This is to ensure that the reader will be able to understand the preventive measures described in the book in a better way once these factors and causes are known.

Genetic Factors

Inheritance Patterns

Genetics can significantly influence the likelihood of developing diabetes. Both Type 1 and Type 2 Diabetes have genetic components, meaning the condition can run in families. The inheritance patterns differ between Type 1 and Type 2 Diabetes. T1DM often appears suddenly and is influenced by a combination of genes and environmental triggers. T2DM tends to develop gradually and can be passed down through multiple generations in a family. Some forms of diabetes, like Maturity Onset Diabetes of the Young (MODY), are caused by a mutation in a single gene (*monogenic*). In contrast, most diabetes cases result from variations in multiple genes (*polygenic*).

Specific Genes Involved

Certain genes have been identified as playing a crucial role in diabetes. For instance, HLA genes are linked to Type 1 Diabetes, and the TCF7L2 gene is associated with Type 2 Diabetes. These genes affect how the body regulates blood sugar and how the immune system functions, which can lead to the development of diabetes. In single-gene types like MODY, mutations alter how the body produces and uses insulin.

Family History

Having a close family member, such as a parent or sibling, with diabetes increases an individual's risk of developing the condition. Studies show that if one has a first-degree relative with diabetes, the risk of developing the disease is significantly higher than someone without such a family history. Hence, knowing one's family's medical history is crucial for assessing the person's risk and taking appropriate preventive measures.

Ethnicity and Genetic Predisposition

Some ethnic groups have higher rates of diabetes. For example, African Americans, Hispanics, Native Americans, and Asians are more likely to develop diabetes. These groups often have genetic factors that make them more susceptible to diabetes. This genetic predisposition can indicate how they should manage their risk and take appropriate preventive measures by following a healthy lifestyle.

<u>Epigenetics</u>

Epigenetics is the study of how lifestyle and environmental factors can change how genes work without altering the DNA sequence. These changes can impact the risk of developing diabetes. Factors like diet, stress, and exposure to toxins can affect the expression of genes, potentially leading to diabetes. Researchers are exploring how epigenetic changes contribute to diabetes, aiming to find new ways to prevent and treat the disease.

Lifestyle Factors (Diet, Physical Activity)

<u>Diet</u>

Eating a diet that is high in calories and sugar can lead to insulin resistance, which is an important factor in the development of T2DM. This type of diet can cause the body to struggle to control blood sugar levels. Consuming too many refined carbohydrates, sugary drinks, and foods with trans fats can increase the risk of diabetes. These foods can spike blood sugar levels and lead to long-term health problems. The importance of a balanced diet cannot be overemphasized. A balanced diet includes whole grains, fruits, vegetables, and lean proteins. These foods help maintain stable blood sugar levels and maintain overall health.

<u>Obesity</u>

Being overweight or obese is strongly linked to insulin resistance, where the body's cells do not respond properly to insulin. This can lead to higher blood sugar levels and an increased risk of T2DM. Many studies show that obesity is one of the major risk factors for developing T2DM. The heavier a person, the higher their risk. Fat stored around the abdomen, known as *visceral fat*, is particularly harmful. It interferes with insulin regulation and can lead to metabolic problems.

Physical Activity

Sedentary habits significantly increase the risk of developing type 2 diabetes. Hence, regular physical activity is crucial for preventing and managing diabetes. Exercise helps the body use insulin more efficiently and improves blood sugar control. When one exercises, the muscles use glucose for energy, which lowers blood sugar levels. Regular activity also helps maintain a healthy weight and reduces insulin resistance. Experts recommend at least 150 minutes of moderate aerobic activity, like walking or cycling, each week. Strength training exercises are also beneficial for maintaining muscle mass and improving metabolism. [See chapter 17 on *Exercise and Physical Activity Plans*].

Sedentary Lifestyle

Prolonged inactivity can lead to weight gain, insulin resistance, and higher blood sugar levels, all of which are major risk factors for type 2 diabetes. Sitting for long periods increases the risk of developing diabetes. A sedentary lifestyle, often linked to certain jobs and daily habits, often leads to poor blood sugar control and weight gain. Jobs that involve sitting for most of the day can contribute to a higher risk of diabetes. Office workers, IT and Tech professionals, call center employees, writers, editors, lawyers, paralegals and drivers are some of the professions more prone to develop T2DM. One should incorporate more movement into one's day by taking regular breaks to stand up, walk around, or do light exercises which can be done even while sitting. Simple actions like taking the stairs instead of the elevator can make a big difference.

Smoking and Alcohol Consumption

Smoking is harmful to many aspects of health, including increasing the risk of insulin resistance and T2DM.

Quitting smoking can significantly improve overall health and reduce diabetes risk. Drinking too much alcohol can lead to high blood sugar levels and affect how the body uses insulin. Moderation is key to maintaining healthy blood sugar levels. Smoking should be avoided altogether, and alcohol consumption should be limited. For those who drink, moderation means up to one drink per day for women and up to two drinks per day for men.

Environmental Factors

Urbanization and Lifestyle Changes

As cities grow and become more modern, people's lifestyles change in ways that can increase the risk of diabetes. Urban living often means more access to unhealthy fast food and processed food, less physical activity, and higher stress levels from busy city life. With modernization, many people tend to eat more processed and fast foods and consume soft drinks, which are high in sugar and unhealthy fats. Additionally, people often become less physically active due to sedentary jobs and conveniences like cars and elevators. The stress of urban living can also contribute to the development of diabetes.

Exposure to Toxins

Certain chemicals in the environment, such as pesticides and hormone-disrupting chemicals, may play a role in developing diabetes. These toxins can interfere with how the body processes insulin and glucose. Scientists are studying how these toxins affect insulin resistance and the function of beta cells, which produce insulin in the pancreas. Understanding these effects can help us learn more about preventing diabetes.

Mark, a 40-year-old jet-setting business executive, was diagnosed with type 2 diabetes mellitus during his yearly medical checkup. Overweight and mostly sedentary, Mark's busy schedule involved frequent travel to distant places and stays in hotels, making it difficult to maintain a healthy lifestyle.

Managing diabetes posed significant challenges for Mark. He needed to monitor his blood sugar levels regularly, which was difficult with his hectic travel schedule. Adopting a balanced diet was another hurdle, as he often relied on restaurant meals and room service. Finding time for regular exercise was also challenging, given his long work hours and constant travel.

Balancing diabetes management with his career required Mark to make substantial lifestyle changes. He had to plan his meals carefully, choosing healthier options even when dining out. He also needed to find ways to incorporate physical activity into his routine, such as using hotel gyms or taking walks between meetings.

Mark's healthcare team advised him on how to manage his condition while traveling, emphasizing the importance of medication adherence, regular blood sugar monitoring, and maintaining a healthy lifestyle. Over time, Mark learned to prioritize his health, making necessary adjustments to his routine to effectively manage his diabetes while continuing to succeed in his career.

Socioeconomic Factors

Socioeconomic status can greatly impact a person's ability to access healthy foods, healthcare, and opportunities for physical activity. Those with lower socioeconomic status often face barriers that can increase their risk of developing diabetes. Studies show that people in the lower socioeconomic strata of society tend to have higher rates of diabetes. This is often due to factors like limited access to nutritious foods, fewer opportunities for regular exercise, and less access to medical care.

Geographical Variations

Diabetes prevalence can vary significantly across different regions and countries. This variation is influenced by factors such as diet, lifestyle, and climate. In some regions, traditional diets and active lifestyles help protect against diabetes, while in others, modern diets high in processed foods and sedentary habits contribute to higher rates of the disease.

Psychosocial Stress

Chronic stress can disrupt the balance of hormones in the body and affect glucose metabolism leading to higher blood sugar levels and an increased risk of diabetes. Learning and practicing stress management techniques, such as relaxation exercises, mindfulness, and regular physical activity, can help reduce the risk of diabetes. Managing stress is an important part of maintaining overall health and preventing various chronic diseases. [see Chapter 14 on *Psychological and Emotional Aspects*].

Other Medical Conditions

High Blood Pressure

High blood pressure (*Hypertension*) is often linked to insulin resistance, which is a major factor in the development of diabetes. When the body becomes resistant to insulin, it can lead to higher blood sugar levels. Having high blood pressure can make managing diabetes more challenging. It increases the risk of complications, such as heart disease and kidney problems, making it important to control both blood pressure and blood sugar levels.

Abnormal Lipid Levels

Lipids are the fats and oils that are needed for a variety of body functions. They are present in blood. Abnormal levels of lipids in the blood are called *Dyslipidemia*. The lipids present in blood are LDL (bad cholesterol), HDL (good cholesterol), and Triglycerides. Abnormal levels of lipids in blood can contribute to the development of diabetes. High levels of bad cholesterol and triglycerides can lead to insulin resistance. [See Chapter 8 on *Complications of Diabetes*].

Polycystic Ovary Syndrome (PCOS)

Polycystic Ovary Syndrome (PCOS) is a condition that affects women's hormone levels. Women with PCOS often have insulin resistance, which increases their risk of developing T2DM. PCOS causes hormonal imbalances that can affect how the body processes glucose, leading to higher blood sugar levels and an increased risk of diabetes.

Gestational Diabetes

Gestational diabetes (GDM) occurs during pregnancy and increases the risk of developing T2DM later in life. Women who have had gestational diabetes need to monitor their blood sugar levels even after pregnancy. During pregnancy, hormonal changes can make it harder for the body to use insulin effectively, leading to gestational diabetes. Managing this condition is important for both mother and baby. [See Chapter 6 on *Gestational Diabetes*].

Chronic Inflammation

Inflammation indicates the body's response to injury or infection. The body releases certain chemicals to trigger an immune response which helps heal the injury or fight the infection. Chronic inflammation in the body can contribute to insulin resistance, which is a key factor in the development of diabetes. Inflammation can interfere with how the body uses insulin, leading to higher blood sugar levels. Certain chemical compounds in the blood, like C-reactive protein, indicate that inflammation is present in the body. High levels of these markers are associated with an increased risk of diabetes.

Other Endocrine Disorders

Certain endocrine disorders, such as Cushing's syndrome (Adrenal gland disease), Acromegaly (Pituitary gland disease), and Hyperthyroidism (Thyroid gland disease), increase the risk of diabetes. These conditions affect hormone levels, which can interfere with how the body processes glucose. These endocrine disorders can disrupt normal glucose metabolism, leading to insulin resistance and higher blood sugar levels, resulting in diabetes.

Medication-Induced Diabetes

Some medications, like corticosteroids, antipsychotics, and beta-blockers, can raise blood sugar levels and increase the risk of diabetes. It is important to manage blood sugar levels carefully if a person is taking these medications. If a person is on medications that affect blood glucose levels, the doctor may provide specific strategies to help manage one's diabetes and minimize the risk of medication-induced diabetes.

Infections and Immune Disorders

Certain viral infections can trigger autoimmune responses that lead to Type 1 Diabetes. These infections can cause the body's immune system to attack insulin-producing cells in the pancreas. Immune disorders can affect the body's ability to manage blood glucose levels, increasing the risk of diabetes. Managing these disorders is important to help control blood sugar levels and prevent complications.

SYMPTOMS AND SIGNS OF DIABETES (T1 & R2DM)

Common Symptoms of Diabetes

The symptoms of Diabetes are common to all types of diabetes. Gestational diabetes may however, present without symptoms and is often detected on routine prenatal blood examination.

Frequent Urination (*Polyuria*)

When blood sugar levels are too high, the kidneys try to remove the excess glucose by producing more urine. This leads to frequent urination. The kidneys work harder to filter out the extra sugar, affecting their function and causing a loss of fluids from the body. Being aware of this symptom can help in diagnosing diabetes early and managing it effectively.

Increased Thirst (*Polydipsia*)

Because the body loses more water through frequent urination, it becomes dehydrated, leading to increased thirst. The person tends to drink more fluids to stay hydrated.

Increased Hunger (*Polyphagia*)

Despite high levels of glucose in the blood, the body's cells cannot use it properly due to a lack of insulin or insulin resistance, making one feel hungry. Without enough insulin, glucose cannot enter the cells, leaving them starved for energy, which triggers hunger.

Unintended Weight Loss

When the body cannot use glucose for energy, it starts breaking down fat and muscle instead, leading to weight loss. This is often seen in people with Type 1 Diabetes and sometimes in those with advanced Type 2 Diabetes.

<u>Fatigue</u>

High blood sugar levels can cause constant tiredness because the body is not able to use glucose effectively for energy. The loss of fluids and muscle tissue also contributes to feeling weak and fatigued.

<u>Blurred Vision</u>

High blood sugar can cause the lenses in the eyes to swell, leading to blurred vision. Blurring can be due to many causes which will be discussed later. If diabetes is not managed well, it can lead to long-term damage to the eyes and vision problems. [See Chapter 8 on *Complications of Diabetes*].

<u>Slow Healing of Wounds</u>

High blood sugar levels can slow down blood circulation and weaken the immune system, making it harder for wounds to heal. Wounds are more prone to infections and complications if blood sugar levels remain high.

<u>Tingling or Numbness</u>

Early signs of nerve damage (*Neuropathy*) due to diabetes include tingling or numbness in the hands and feet. Over time, high blood sugar, if not controlled, can cause significant damage to the nerves.

<u>Recurrent Infections</u>

High blood sugar can weaken the immune system, making the body more susceptible to infections. People with diabetes are more likely to get infections like urinary tract infections, yeast infections, and skin infections.

<u>Dark Patches of Skin</u> (*Acanthosis Nigricans*)

Dark, velvety patches of skin often appear in body folds and creases. These patches are often a sign of insulin resistance and can be an early indicator of diabetes or prediabetes.

DIAGNOSIS OF DIABETES (T1 & T2DM)

The following tests are done for diagnosis of Types 1 and 2 diabetes mellitus.

Fasting Blood Glucose

The main diagnosis of diabetes is made by checking the blood sugar of the patient. For initial diagnosis, the doctor draws blood from a vein in the arm and the blood is then subjected to centrifuging where the liquid part of the blood is separated. This is called *Plasma*. The glucose is estimated in plasma and is called the Plasma Glucose. This gives the value of the amount of glucose in blood. When blood is drawn from the tip of the finger by a finger stick, it estimates the amount of glucose in blood in the capillaries of the finger. Glucose in blood or plasma is usually expressed in milligrams per deciliter (mg/dL) of blood or as millimoles per liter (mmol/L).

The amount of glucose in whole blood is 12% less than the value in plasma. But for practical purposes, this is not of much importance.

Postprandial Blood Glucose Test

Post prandial means after a meal. The post prandial test measures the blood sugar level exactly *two hours* after having eaten a meal to see how the body handles the sugar from the meal.

If the blood sugar level is less than 140 mg/dL (7.8 mmol/L), it is considered normal. If the blood sugar level is between 140 and 199 mg/dL (7.8-11.0 mmol/L), it means that the person has *Prediabetes*, which is a warning sign for potential future diabetes. If the blood sugar level is 200 mg/dL (11.1 mmol/L) or higher, it indicates that the person has diabetes. [See **Table 1**].

HbA1C Test

Another test for diabetes is the estimation of *Glycated Hemoglobin* or *HbA1C* in blood. *Hemoglobin* (**Hb**) is the protein found in red blood cells. This carries oxygen to various tissues in the body. The glucose in blood combines with Hb to form a compound called *Glycated Hemoglobin* or HbA1C or A1C. The amount of HbA1C in blood is directly proportional to the amount of glucose in blood. When glucose levels rise, A1c rises. The glucose is irreversibly bound to the Hb and remains so for 2 -3 months. Hence HbA1C reflects glucose levels over an average of three months. Hence when the blood sugar is high for long periods, the value of HbA1C also is high. Daily fluctuations of blood glucose do not alter the HbA1C and hence, the values give us a measure of the average blood glucose over three months. This is a simple test which does not require fasting blood. HbA1C is expressed as a percentage. The normal HbA1C in an individual is below 5.7%.

The advantages of testing A1C:

- Reflects chronic rise in blood glucose.
- Reflects future complications.
- Fasting is not necessary for a test.
- Helps plan treatment and assess progress and efficacy of treatment.
- Cost effective test – frequent testing not needed.
- Repeat testing is not needed if found high – to diagnose diabetes.

<u>Limitations of HbA1c Test</u>

The HbA1C test is not without some limitations. Some factors can affect the accuracy of the HbA1c test. For example, if one has certain blood disorders like *Sickle Cell Anemia* or if a person has had significant blood loss or *anemia*, the test results might not be accurate. There can be slight differences in HbA1c levels among different ethnic groups, which can sometimes lead to variations in test results.

Random Blood Glucose Test

This test measures the blood sugar level at any random time of the day, no matter when the person last ate. A blood sample is taken whenever one visits the clinic. If the blood sugar level is 200 mg/dL (11.1 mmol/L) or higher, and there are symptoms of diabetes like frequent urination, excessive thirst, or unexplained weight loss, it suggests diabetes. Always, two tests on two separate occasions are done before a diagnosis of diabetes is made.

The table below gives the normal values and those above which diabetes is diagnosed. (**Table 1**).

Result	Plasma Glucose (mg/dL)	Plasma Glucose (mmol/L)	HbA1C (%)	Diagnosis
Fasting Pl. Glu	Less than 100	Less than 5.6	Below 5.7	**Normal**
Fasting Pl. Glu	Between 100 – 125	Between 5.6 – 6.9	Between 5.7 – 6.4	**Prediabetes**
Fasting Pl. Glu	Above 126	Above 7	Above 6.5	**Diabetes mellitus**

Table 1: Normal and Abnormal Values of Blood Sugar

A correlation between the values of **HbA1C** and **Average Blood glucose** and **Average Plasma Glucose** over a 3-month period is given below. (**Table 2**).

HbA1c (%)	5	6	7	8	9	10	12	14
Blood Glucose (mg/dL)	97	126	154	183	212	240	298	355
Plasma Glucose (mg/dL)	100	140	170	210	240	280	350	420

Table 2: HbA1C and Average Blood Sugar

Oral Glucose Tolerance Test

Another test is the Oral Glucose Tolerance Test (OGTT). Here the individual is given 75 grams of glucose orally as a drink and the blood is tested after 2hours. If it is above 200 mg/dL (11.1 mmol/L) diabetes is diagnosed.

Additional Tests

Whenever a diagnosis of diabetes is made an additional group of tests are also done along with it to detect any associated abnormalities. These tests are *Serum Lipid Profile* to detect the levels of various fats in blood, *Liver Function Tests* to know the status of the liver and a careful measurement of the person's Blood Pressure.

A Urine Routine test is always done along with the blood tests. Glucose may be detected in urine. In addition chemicals named *Ketones* may be detected if blood sugar is uncontrolled. Involvement of kidneys may show protein in urine. These will be discussed later in the appropriate sections.

Other additional tests are ordered only if the physician suspects any other abnormality or others causes of diabetes as already discussed above. In Type 1 Diabetes the additional tests needed will be discussed separately.

In addition to these tests, the physician also assesses for any changes indicating complications like involvement of Kidneys, Eyes, Heart and Nervous system by ordering appropriate tests as he deems appropriate. These tests are required when the physician finds any clinical changes suggestive of involvement of other organs.

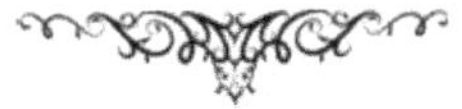

Chapter 6 - GESTATIONAL DIABETES

Gestational Diabetes is a type of diabetes that develops during pregnancy, typically in the second or third trimester. It occurs when the body cannot produce enough insulin to meet the increased demands of pregnancy, leading to high blood sugar levels. Risk factors include being overweight, having a family history of diabetes, being over 25 years old, or having had Gestational Diabetes in a previous pregnancy.

Many women with Gestational Diabetes do not experience noticeable symptoms, which is why routine screening, usually between 24 and 28 weeks of pregnancy, is crucial. If diagnosed, it is important to manage blood sugar levels through diet, exercise, and sometimes medication, to ensure a healthy pregnancy and reduce the risk of complications for both mother and baby. Patient education is vital, as effective management can help prevent the development of Type 2 diabetes later in life for both mother and child. These points are discussed in this chapter.

It is reported that about 8.3% of pregnancies in the US are diagnosed with GDM each year [2021].

Causes and Risk Factors

Various causes and Risk Factors have been identified in the development of GDM.

1. <u>Hormonal Changes</u>.

The placenta located in the uterus produces several hormones during pregnancy, such as human placental lactogen (hPL), estrogen, and progesterone. These hormones are essential for the development of the fetus. However, these hormones can interfere with the normal actions of insulin. Hence the body tends to produce more insulin to maintain normal blood glucose levels.

Many changes occur in the mother's body during pregnancy. Development of resistance to the action of insulin is one such change. The cells in the body become less responsive to insulin resulting in more insulin being produced by the pancreas to keep the blood glucose normal. However, if the pancreas fails to produce enough insulin to overcome this resistance, the patient develops diabetes.

2. <u>Genetic Factors</u>

Women with a family history of diabetes, in parents or siblings have a higher risk of developing gestational diabetes. This indicates that certain genetic factors may influence the way insulin is produced or utilized in the body. These genetic traits affect insulin secretion and glucose metabolism, causing some women to be more susceptible to developing GDM.

3. <u>Lifestyle Factors</u>

Obese women have a higher chance of developing GDM. Excess body fat, particularly around the tummy, often leads to insulin resistance. A sedentary lifestyle without adequate physical activity also worsens this condition by reducing the body's ability to use insulin effectively.

The diet of the individual also contributes to the development of GDM. Diets high in refined sugars, low in fiber and high in unhealthy fats, lead to weight gain and insulin resistance. Eating nutrient-poor, calorie-dense foods also increase the risk of developing GDM. A balanced diet rich in whole grains, fruits, vegetables, and lean proteins is crucial for maintaining healthy blood sugar levels during pregnancy.

4. <u>Other Risk Factors</u>

Maternal age is a major risk factor for developing GDM. It increases linearly with age. Women over the age of 30 are at a higher risk of developing gestational diabetes, with the risk increasing significantly for those over 35. As one ages, metabolism and insulin resistance tend to increase. Women who had gestational diabetes in previous pregnancies are at a higher risk of recurrence in subsequent pregnancies.

Polycystic Ovary Syndrome (PCOS) is a disorder characterized by irregular menstrual periods, excess androgen levels, and multiple cysts in the ovaries. Women with this condition are prone to insulin resistance, and hence to gestational diabetes. The hormonal disturbances associated with PCOS interfere with normal insulin function and glucose metabolism.

Understanding these causes and risk factors allows for better screening, prevention, and management strategies. Regular prenatal check-ups, maintaining a healthy lifestyle, and early intervention can help manage gestational diabetes effectively, ensuring a safe pregnancy and delivery.

<u>**Symptoms of Gestational Diabetes**</u>

The woman with GDM is often does not have any noticeable symptoms. Hence, routine screening during pregnancy is important. Gestational diabetes can go undiagnosed if not looked for. This may lead to complications for both the mother and the baby. When symptoms do occur, they are often like those with other types of diabetes and include increased thirst, frequent urination, fatigue, and blurred vision. These symptoms may be attributed to normal pregnancy changes, and hence GDM may be missed.

Linda, a 23-year-old first-time expectant mother, was diagnosed with gestational diabetes mellitus (GDM) during her first prenatal checkup. The diagnosis surprised her, as she had no prior history of diabetes. Managing her blood sugar levels became a primary concern throughout her pregnancy. Linda had to monitor her glucose levels regularly, adhere to a strict diet, and incorporate regular exercise into her routine. She also needed to take insulin injections, which she found challenging and stressful.

The psychological burden of GDM was significant for Linda. She worried about the health of her baby and felt anxious about the possibility of complications, such as preeclampsia or needing a cesarean section if the baby was large. Postpartum, Linda faced the challenge of maintaining healthy blood sugar levels to reduce her risk of developing type 2 diabetes in the future. She also needed to ensure that she can breastfeed effectively, as GDM could impact milk production.

Linda's baby might face challenges as well. There was an increased risk of being born prematurely, having a higher birth weight, or experiencing low blood sugar levels shortly after birth. In the long term, the baby may have a higher risk of developing obesity or type 2 diabetes. Linda's healthcare team closely monitored both her and her baby, providing guidance to manage these risks effectively.

<u>Screening and Diagnostic Criteria</u>

Screening for gestational diabetes typically is done between 24 and 28 weeks of pregnancy. This is the period when the placenta produces large amounts of hormones which can cause insulin resistance. Early detection is hence essential to manage and reduce potential risks associated with the condition. For women with high-risk factors as discussed before, screening may be conducted earlier in the pregnancy and often repeated later.

<u>Fasting Blood Glucose Test</u>: This test measures blood sugar levels after an overnight fast of at least 8 hours. It is less commonly used alone for diagnosing gestational diabetes but can be part of an initial screening. A fasting blood glucose level of 92 mg/dL (5.1 mmol/L) or higher may indicate gestational diabetes. Note that the blood glucose levels to diagnose GDM are slightly lower than that for non-pregnant adults.

<u>Random Blood Glucose Test</u>: This test measures blood sugar levels regardless of when the last meal was consumed. It can be used as a preliminary test. A random blood glucose level of 200 mg/dL (11.1 mmol/L) or higher suggests diabetes, but further testing with OGTT is usually required.

<u>Oral Glucose Tolerance Test (OGTT)</u>: The OGTT is the primary diagnostic test for gestational diabetes. It involves fasting overnight (8 hours) and then drinking a solution containing 75 gms. of glucose. Blood samples are taken at fasting, and then at one, two, and sometimes three hours after consuming the glucose. GDM is diagnosed if the blood levels are as follows:

- Fasting Blood Glucose Level: 92 mg/dL (5.1 mmol/L) or higher.

- One-Hour Blood Glucose Level: 180 mg/dL (10.0 mmol/L) or higher after one hour.

- Two-Hour Blood Glucose Level: 153 mg/dL (8.5 mmol/L) or higher after two hours.

- Three-Hour Blood Glucose Level (if measured): 140 mg/dL (7.8 mmol/L) or higher after three hours.

Management of GDM

Management During Pregnancy

Monitoring Blood Glucose: Blood glucose must be regularly monitored in GDM. Blood sugar levels must be checked multiple times daily to ensure that blood sugar levels remain within the expected range to reduce the risk of complications.

The target blood glucose levels for women with gestational diabetes are set lower than for non-pregnant women with diabetes. Hence, a fasting blood glucose level of less than 95 mg/dL (5.3 mmol/L), and one-hour postprandial levels of less than 140 mg/dL (7.8 mmol/L) or two-hour postprandial levels of less than 120 mg/dL (6.7 mmol/L) are the usual goals to be attained.

Nutritional Counseling: A balanced diet to meet the nutritional needs of pregnancy and at the same time maintaining blood glucose levels is needed. Eating three small meals and two to three snacks daily spreading the carbohydrate intake throughout the day is important. Complex carbohydrates, fiber-rich foods, lean proteins, and healthy fats should be consumed.

One should learn to count carbohydrates to manage blood sugar levels. The Glycemic Index (GI) of foods should be known. [See Chapter 18 on *Nutritional Recipes & Meal Plans*]. Foods with a low to moderate GI are preferred as they cause a slow rise in blood sugar levels.

Physical Activity: Regular physical activity improves insulin sensitivity and controls blood glucose levels. Pregnant women are encouraged moderate exercise, such as walking, swimming, or prenatal yoga, for at least 30 minutes most days of the week.

Insulin Therapy: If diet and exercise fail to control sugar levels, insulin therapy is needed. Insulin is safe for both the mother and the baby and helps keep blood glucose levels within the expected range. The type and dosage of insulin are determined based on the individual's blood glucose patterns. Insulin is administered through injections or through insulin pumps.

The effectiveness of insulin treatment is monitored by frequently checking blood sugar. Insulin requirements may change as pregnancy progresses. The physician will advise on the change in dose of insulin depending on the levels of blood sugar.

Postpartum Considerations

Long-Term Risk: Those with GDM are at a higher risk of developing T2DM later in life. Up to 50% of women with GDM will develop T2DM within 5 to 10 years after delivery.

Some factors influencing the risk of developing diabetes in future are the degree of insulin resistance present during pregnancy, obesity, and a family history of diabetes. The risk is reduced by maintaining a healthy weight and lifestyle.

Postpartum Monitoring: The American Diabetes Association recommends a 75-gram oral glucose tolerance test (OGTT) at 6-12 weeks after delivery. Regular monitoring should continue, especially if the initial postpartum test indicates impaired glucose regulation.

Lifestyle Modifications: A healthy lifestyle must be continued after delivery to prevent the development of T2DM.

This includes a balanced diet, regular physical activity, and maintaining a healthy weight. Breastfeeding is encouraged, as it can help weight loss and improve glucose metabolism.

<u>Regular Medical Follow-Up:</u> Women with GDM must be on a regular medical follow up with their healthcare provider and monitor glucose levels to check for development of diabetes.

Effective management of gestational diabetes during pregnancy and proactive care after delivery are important for ensuring the long-term health of both the mother and the baby.

Chapter 7 - TYPE 1 DIABETES MELLITUS
Causes, Risk Factors, Symptoms & Diagnosis

*Type 1 Diabetes (**T1DM**) is an autoimmune condition where the body's immune system mistakenly attacks the insulin-producing cells in the pancreas. Unlike Type 2, which is often related to lifestyle factors, Type 1 is primarily influenced by genetic and environmental factors. This chapter will discuss the causes and risk factors associated with T1DM, providing insights into what triggers this autoimmune response. Understanding the symptoms—such as sudden weight loss, extreme thirst, and frequent urination—is crucial for early detection, especially since T1DM often presents suddenly and can quickly lead to serious complications if not diagnosed promptly. This chapter also covers the diagnostic processes, including blood tests and other evaluations that help confirm T1DM.*

Type 1 diabetes (T1DM), previously known as *Juvenile Diabetes* or *Insulin Dependent Diabetes mellitus* (IDDM), is a chronic condition where the body is unable to produce insulin due to the autoimmune destruction of insulin-producing beta cells in the pancreas. This results in increased blood glucose levels, requiring lifelong management with insulin treatment. Unlike type 2 diabetes, which is often associated with lifestyle factors, T1DM is primarily influenced by genetic and autoimmune factors, with environmental triggers which also play a role in its genesis. Getting to know the causes and risk factors of T1DM is important for developing preventive strategies and improving management of the disease.

CAUSES AND RISK FACTORS FOR T1DM

1. <u>Genetic Factors</u>:   Certain genes increase the risk of developing T1DM. These genes are involved in immune system regulation, and their variations can predispose an individual to various types of autoimmune diseases, including T1DM.

The family history of T1DM is a major risk factor. If a first-degree relative (parent or sibling) has type 1 diabetes, the risk of developing the disease increases significantly. Siblings of individuals with T1DM have about a 6% risk, while children of affected fathers have an 8% risk, and children of affected mothers have a 3% risk according to various studies. If both parents have diabetes, the risk is 30% (6 times) compared to a person whose parents have no diabetes.

The inappropriate immune response against the body's own tissues, as discussed below, is also genetically mediated. This predisposition is a key factor in causing the disease.

2. <u>Autoimmune Response</u>:   In T1DM the body's immune system mistakenly targets and destroys the insulin-producing beta cells in the pancreas. This destruction of beta cells occurs gradually over time. Initially, there may be sufficient beta cell function to maintain normal glucose levels,

but as the immune-mediated destruction progresses, insulin production decreases, leading to high blood sugar levels. By the time clinical symptoms appear, about 80-90% of beta cells have already been destroyed.

3. <u>Environmental Factors</u>: Several studies have suggested that viral infections could trigger the onset of T1DM in genetically predisposed individuals suggesting a possible causal link. Early dietary exposures have also been proposed as potential risk factors. For instance, early introduction of cow's milk and a lack of breastfeeding have been associated with an increased risk of developing T1DM. The exact mechanisms are not known, but it is hypothesized that these dietary factors may adversely influence the development of the immune system in infancy.

4. <u>Geographical and Ethnic Factors</u>: The incidence of T1DM varies significantly by geography, with higher prevalence rates in Northern European countries and lower rates in Asian countries. This suggests that environmental factors, possibly related to climate, infections, or lifestyle, may influence the risk of developing the disease. The condition is more common in Native American, African American, Hispanic, Asian American and Pacific islanders in the US than in the general population.

Significant research efforts are still ongoing to unravel the underlying causes of T1DM and developing preventive strategies. The genetic, immunological, and environmental factors involved in the disease process are being studied. Many theories are also expounded. One theory is the 'Hygiene hypothesis,' which suggests that reduced exposure to infectious agents in early childhood may lead to an underdeveloped immune system that is more prone to autoimmune diseases. This hypothesis is supported by epidemiological data showing higher rates of T1DM in cleaner, more industrialized environments as in the west than in the countries in the east.

SYMPTOMS OF T1DM

- Frequent Urination (*Polyuria*) is a common symptom. Increased blood glucose levels lead to excess glucose in the urine, which draws more water from the body, causing frequent urination.

- Excessive Thirst (*Polydipsia*) occurs because of increased urine output. As the body tends to become dehydrated, the person feels excessive thirst to compensate for the fluid loss.

- Extreme Hunger (*Polyphagia*) is another important symptom. Despite high blood glucose levels, the body's cells are starved for energy due to a lack of insulin, leading to increased hunger as the body tries to get more glucose.

- Unexplained Weight Loss occurs as the body is unable to use glucose for energy and hence it breaks down fat and muscle tissue for fuel leading to weight loss.

- Fatigue and weakness occur as glucose does not enter the cells in adequate amounts and hence the body lacks the necessary energy.

- Blurred Vision is because the high blood glucose levels cause the lenses of the eyes to swell, leading to blurring of vision.

- Slow-Healing Sores and frequent Infections are seen as high blood glucose levels impair the immune system, impairing the healing of wounds. The person becomes prone to repeated infections.

- Ketones are detected in the urine as the body begins to breakdown fat for energy. Ketones are the byproduct of fat breakdown which can accumulate in the urine and indicate diabetic ketoacidosis - a dangerous complication in T1DM.

In children and adolescents, T1DM often has an abrupt onset, with symptoms appearing over a few days or weeks. Early recognition of symptoms is important to prevent severe complications such as diabetic ketoacidosis.

In adults, T1DM can develop more gradually and may initially be mistaken for T2DM due to the overlapping symptoms. Misdiagnosis can delay appropriate treatment, highlighting the importance of accurate and timely diagnosis.

David, a 14-year-old high school freshman, was recently diagnosed with type 1 diabetes. He now faced the challenge of regularly monitoring his blood sugar, which involved frequent finger pricks and calculating insulin doses. Despite his efforts, he occasionally got high blood sugar levels that affected his concentration and low blood sugar episodes that caused dizziness and shakiness.

At school, David felt self-conscious about checking his blood sugar and administering insulin in front of his peers. Some classmates' curiosity and insensitive comments made him uncomfortable, and he struggled with not being able to eat the same snacks and treats as his friends. Social activities, like birthday parties and sleepovers, added to his anxiety about managing his condition.

With support from his family and healthcare team, David learned to manage his diabetes more confidently. His school created a supportive environment, and his friends gradually became more understanding and helpful. Over time, David balanced his health needs with his social life and school activities, gaining confidence and learning to communicate his needs effectively.

DIAGNOSIS OF T1DM

By far, the diagnostic values of blood glucose in T1DM are the same as for T2DM. These have been discussed all ready. Briefly they are given below.

- Fasting blood glucose levels of ≥126 mg/dL (7.0 mmol/L) on two separate occasions.
- Random blood glucose levels of ≥200 mg/dL (11.1 mmol/L) with symptoms of hyperglycemia.
- Blood glucose level of ≥200 mg/dL (11.1 mmol/L) two hours after consuming a 75 g glucose-containing beverage.
- Glycated hemoglobin (HbA1c) level of ≥6.5%.

Autoantibody Testing

Autoantibodies against *Glutamic Acid Decarboxylase* (GADA), *insulinoma-associated antigen-2* (IA-2A), *insulin* (IAA), and the newly identified *Zinc Transporter 8* (ZnT8A) serve as some of the most reliable biomarkers for detecting autoimmune diabetes in both children and adults. The test detects the presence of autoantibodies that attack pancreatic beta cells, confirming an autoimmune cause for diabetes. Autoantibody testing helps differentiate T1DM from other types, confirming the autoimmune nature of the disease and guiding appropriate treatment strategies.

C-Peptide Test

Measurement of C-peptide levels, which are released in equal amounts to insulin, indicates the level of insulin produced by the pancreas. This helps to assess residual beta-cell function. Low C-peptide levels indicate T1DM, showing that there is only minimal or no residual beta-cell function. Low or undetectable C-peptide levels confirm the diagnosis of

T1DM, differentiating it from T2DM, where C-peptide levels may remain normal or elevated.

DIFFERENTIATING TYPE 1 FROM TYPE 2 DIABETES

- T1DM is often of rapid onset, often in children and adolescents, with symptoms of high blood sugar levels and ketosis.
- T2DM is of gradual onset, typically in adults, associated with obesity, insulin resistance, and less pronounced symptoms.
- T1DM requires insulin therapy from the onset, while T2DM may initially be managed with lifestyle changes and oral medications. Insulin may be required only late in the disease.

Understanding the symptoms and diagnostic criteria for T1DM is essential for early detection and effective management. Seeking prompt medical evaluation can prevent severe complications and improve the quality of life for individuals with T1DM.

Chapter 8 - COMPLICATIONS OF DIABETES

In this chapter, we will describe the various complications that can arise from diabetes, affecting multiple parts of the body. Understanding these complications is crucial for prevention and early intervention. The acute complications like Hypoglycemia, Severe hyperglycemia and Diabetic Ketoacidosis are discussed first. We will discuss cardiovascular issues, including heart disease and stroke, which are common among diabetic patients. Kidney problems, or diabetic nephropathy, will also be covered, highlighting the importance of regular screening. Eye complications, such as diabetic retinopathy, can lead to vision loss if not managed properly. Skin conditions and infections, prevalent in diabetics, will be explained, along with preventive measures. Foot complications, like ulcers and infections, are another critical area due to poor circulation and nerve damage. By learning about these potential complications, you can take proactive steps in managing your diabetes and maintaining overall health.

The complications of diabetes can be either acute and abrupt in onset or chronic when they occur in long standing diabetes and develop over a period.

ACUTE COMPLICATIONS

Acute complications are those that can occur at any time and are often sudden in onset. *Hypoglycemia, Diabetic Ketoacidosis* and *Hyperosmolar Hyperglycemic State* are the common acute complications. They are discussed in detail below.

HYPOGLYCEMIA

Hypoglycemia, commonly known as low blood sugar, occurs when blood glucose levels drop below **70 mg/dL.** This is a common complication which can happen for various reasons, and it is very important that every patient and his/her caregiver knows about it. Hypoglycemia can occur in both types of diabetes. Teachers and the school authorities should be aware of this if they have children with diabetes in their school.

Some of the causes why hypoglycemia occurs are given below.

- One of the common reasons why this occurs is taking too much insulin or taking insulin and not eating food on time.
- Skipping meals or not eating adequate food can also cause hypoglycemia.
- Drinking excess alcohol, especially on an empty stomach, can lead to hypoglycemia.
- Intense physical activity can use up a lot of glucose, leading to a sudden lowering of blood glucose levels.
- Going on a diet without adjusting one's medications can lead to hypoglycemia.

- Not taking mid-morning snacks or a bedtime snack can lead to hypoglycemia at lunch time or midnight.
- Severe liver or kidney disease can cause hypoglycemia.
- Eating disorders, especially in adolescents, may lead to hypoglycemic episodes.

<u>Symptoms</u>

When blood sugar levels begin to drop, the individual gets early warning signs. Feeling shaky, sweating more than usual, feeling anxious, yawning and excess hunger are some such early symptoms. The person may feel irritable and get unusually angry. Some may get hypoglycemia at night while sleeping and it may go unrecognized. The patient may have nightmares or profuse sweating which may be noticed by the partner or by the mother in the case of children. Rarely, seizures may occur during sleep. Palpitations may occur as hypoglycemia can trigger irregular heartbeats (*Arrhythmia*).

When hypoglycemia becomes more severe it can lead to confusion, difficulty in thinking clearly, lack of concentration, disorientation, seizures, and loss of consciousness. Often the patient becomes irritable and prone to anger. Elderly patients who develop recurrent hypoglycemia may develop dementia subsequently. Recognizing these symptoms early and taking prompt action is crucial to prevent serious complications.

<u>Mechanisms</u>

As we have seen already, the body uses insulin and other hormones to keep blood sugar levels within the normal range. Insulin lowers blood sugar, while hormones like glucagon and epinephrine raise it when it gets too low. When blood sugar drops too low, it can have an adverse effect on the brain, which relies solely on glucose for its metabolism. Without enough glucose, the brain fails to function properly, leading to symptoms like confusion, seizures and coma. The body tries to compensate for hypoglycemia by increasing glucose production by releasing glucagon, adrenaline and other hormones. While glucagon breaks down glycogen into glucose, adrenaline in addition to raising glucose produces the symptoms like sweating, anxiety, increased heart rate and tremors.

<u>Management</u>

The first step in treating hypoglycemia is to raise blood sugar levels quickly by eating or drinking something. This could be glucose tablets or a sugary drink like juice. Ideally, 4 glucose tablets (4 gms/tablet), 15 grams of sugar (1 tablespoon) or a cup of fruit juice or milk suffices. For long-term management, however, it is important to adjust the medications and monitor blood sugar levels frequently. A regular eating schedule to keep blood sugar stable should be followed. Teaching the patient and caregiver(s) to recognize the symptoms of hypoglycemia and knowing how to respond immediately is important.

Prevention of hypoglycemia involves learning how to balance food intake, medication, and physical activity to avoid sudden drop in blood sugar levels. Being aware of the symptoms and knowing how to take immediate action if hypoglycemia occurs is equally important. Eating a snack every hour is important if one is doing severe exercise like marathon running, hiking or playing soccer. Meals should be eaten soon after injecting insulin.

<u>Risks and Consequences</u>

Hypoglycemia should not be taken lightly. Severe hypoglycemia can lead to dangerous situations, such as accidents or injuries, because it can impair judgment and coordination. Hence patients prone to hypoglycemia should be careful while driving and handling machinery. It can also trigger serious health events like cardiac problems. Frequent episodes of hypoglycemia can affect a person's quality of life and can cause fear and anxiety about when the next episode might happen. This in turn can lead to stress and impact the mental well-being of the individual. Careful management of blood sugar levels helps reduce these risks and improve overall health and quality of life.

DIABETIC KETOACIDOSIS (DKA)

Diabetic Ketoacidosis (DKA) is a serious and potentially life-threatening complication. It occurs when there is very high blood sugar and inadequate insulin to tackle these high levels. The body begins to break down fat and this leads to the generation of chemicals collectively named *Ketones*. These chemicals are *Acetone, Acetoacetic acid* and *Beta hydroxy butyric acid*. These cause the blood to become too acidic. This dangerous situation can develop suddenly and needs immediate medical attention and hospitalization. DKA is primarily caused by a significant lack of insulin in the body. DKA occurs more commonly in T1DM compared to T2DM.

DKA can happen due to various reasons, like not taking enough insulin, having an infection or illness which increases the insulin requirement, or missing insulin doses. It can also be triggered by stress or other medical conditions that increase the body's demand for insulin.

The *ketones* produced are acidic chemicals which cause the blood to become too acidic, leading to a condition known as *Acidosis*. Acidosis can disrupt the normal balance of electrolytes and fluids in the body, causing further complications and making the person acutely ill.

<u>Symptoms</u>

The early symptoms of DKA are extreme thirst and frequent urination. The person is dehydrated with loss of skin turgor, sunken eyes and cracked, dry lips. These are signs that the body is trying to get rid of excess glucose through urine. The tongue may be covered with thick white fur. High blood sugar levels are also an early indicator. As the condition worsens, more severe symptoms like nausea, vomiting and abdominal pain develop. The patient's breath has a distinct fruity smell. This is due to the ketones which are present in the exhaled air. The patient's breathing becomes rapid and often the patient becomes confused. The patient may become apathetic and develop delirium. He can lose consciousness. DKA is most commonly seen in T1DM but can also occur in T2DM.

Diagnosis

DKA is diagnosed by blood tests. Blood glucose levels are high. Ketones are detected in the urine and blood. Other tests in blood indicate acidosis.

Treatment

Treating DKA requires immediate hospitalization and medical intervention. The patient must be rehydrated rapidly with intravenous fluids, as they are often severely dehydrated. Insulin is started immediately to lower blood glucose levels and prevent the production of ketones. Along with insulin, it is important to replace other electrolytes like Sodium, Potassium and Chloride to restore the body's balance and address any underlying causes, such as infections or missed insulin doses. The cause as to why the patient developed DKA should be probed, and appropriate action taken.

Prevention

Preventing DKA involves careful and regular monitoring of blood glucose levels. It is also important to follow insulin therapy as prescribed and to recognize and treat any infections or illnesses promptly. The patient and the caregiver(s) should be made aware of the signs and symptoms of high blood sugar and ketosis.

This can help in taking quick action to prevent DKA from developing. Educating patients and their families about the importance of adherence to treatment and how to respond to early warning signs can significantly reduce the risk of this dangerous complication.

The school authorities too should be informed about the child's health if he is having diabetes, so that any change in behavior or abnormal symptoms is promptly recognized and appropriate action taken.

HYPEROSMOLAR HYPERGLYCEMIC STATE (HHS)

Hyperosmolar Hyperglycemic State (HHS) is a serious complication that occurs when blood sugar levels become extremely high without significant ketosis. This condition needs immediate medical attention. As in DKA, HHS can also be triggered by various factors. Some of these are:

- Severe infections like Respiratory and Urinary infections may trigger HHS.
- Poor management of Type 2 Diabetes and failure to take diabetic medications. This can happen with elderly people living alone who forget to take their medications or suffer from unrecognized infections.
- Certain medications like Thiazide diuretics, Corticosteroids, certain Antipsychotics, and others like Beta-blockers, Dilantin, and Statins which are used to treat high cholesterol.
- Cardiovascular problems like Stroke, Angina pectoris, and Heart Attack can also cause HHS which release hormones like Adrenaline and Steroids which increase the blood glucose levels.
- Dehydration by itself can lead to HHS.
- HHS is most commonly seen in patients with type 2 diabetes. But may occur in type 1 diabetes also.

The extremely high blood sugar levels cause the body to become severely dehydrated because the kidneys try to get rid of the excess sugar by increasing urine production leading to a significant loss of fluids. As a result, the plasma, or the liquid part of the blood, becomes very concentrated. Unlike DKA, HHS does not result in significant ketone production because there is still some insulin present in the body. The presence of insulin prevents the body from breaking down fat into ketones, which is why ketosis does not occur prominently in HHS.

<u>Symptoms</u>

Early symptoms of HHS include extreme thirst and frequent urination just as in DKA. Blood sugar levels will be extremely high during this stage. If the condition worsens, severe symptoms develop. These are dehydration, which causes dry skin and a dry mouth. The patient has sunken eyes and a rapid pulse. Leg cramps often occur. Confusion, seizures, and even coma can occur in severe cases as the high concentration of sugar in the blood affects brain function.

<u>Diagnosis</u>

A detailed clinical assessment by the physician will evaluate dehydration and the neurological status. This helps in understanding the severity of dehydration and any effects on brain function, which is crucial for proper diagnosis and treatment. HHS is diagnosed with blood tests. These show a very high blood glucose level. The values are often above 600 mg/dL. A high serum osmolality indicating a high concentration of substances in the blood, and an absence of significant ketones is seen.

<u>Treatment</u>

Immediate hospitalization is needed in HHS. Aggressive rehydration is begun immediately with intravenous fluids, to restore the lost fluids. Insulin therapy is essential to lower blood glucose levels quickly. It is given as frequent bolus injections or as a continuous infusion. Alongside insulin, it is necessary to correct any electrolyte imbalances that have occurred due to dehydration. Monitoring for other associated complications like blood clots (*Thrombosis*) and infections is also a vital part of the treatment process.

<u>Prevention</u>

Preventing HHS involves regular monitoring of blood glucose levels and staying well-hydrated to prevent severe dehydration. Following the diabetes management plan given by the physician and seeking prompt medical attention when blood sugar levels are high significantly reduces the risk of HHS. Educating patients about the importance of proper blood sugar control, recognizing early signs, and maintaining good hydration can help prevent this dangerous complication. Infections should be diagnosed early, and treatment instituted. The elderly living alone should have a relative or a caregiver check on them frequently.

CHRONIC COMPLICATIONS

CARDIOVASCULAR DISEASE (CVD)

People with diabetes have a much higher risk of developing heart disease, stroke, and peripheral artery disease compared to those without diabetes. This is because diabetes can cause many changes in the body that increase the risk of these conditions. One of the main reasons for this increased risk is high blood sugar levels. Consistently high blood sugar can cause damage to blood vessels and nerves. Other factors that increase the cardiovascular risk in diabetics are high blood pressure (*Hypertension*), high levels of blood cholesterol and other fats in the blood (*Dyslipidemia*), and ongoing inflammation. Together, these factors can significantly raise the chances of having a heart attack, stroke, or other heart-related problems.

When blood glucose levels remain high for a long period, it tends to damage the walls of blood vessels. This results in fatty deposits to build up inside the walls of the arteries, a condition known as *Atherosclerosis*. These plaques can cause narrowing of the blood vessels to the brain causing Stroke, blood vessels to the heart (*Coronary Arteries*) causing Heart Attack and those to the legs causing blood supply to be affected. (**Fig 1**). When these *plaques* enlarge, they can reduce blood flow or even block the blood vessel completely, leading to heart attacks or strokes. Insulin resistance, a common issue in people with T2DM, can also contribute to cardiovascular problems. When blood vessels to the lower limbs are affected, the circulation to the limbs may suffer leading to ulcers in the feet and occasionally gangrene which may necessitate amputation of the limb.

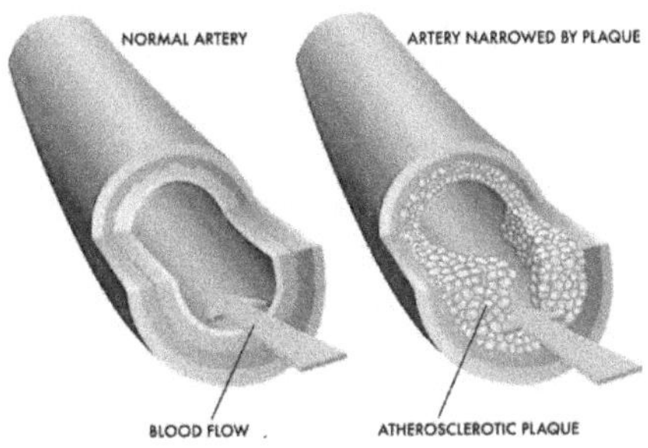

Fig 1. Shows a Normal artery and one narrowed by a Plaque.

Insulin resistance increases blood lipids, or fats, leading to higher levels of bad cholesterol (*Low Density Lipoproteins* or **LDL**) and lower levels of good cholesterol (*High Density Lipoproteins* or **HDL**) in blood. It can also affect how the body regulates blood pressure, making it more likely for high blood pressure to develop. These changes increase the risk of heart disease and stroke.

Symptoms

Symptoms of heart disease are chest pain or discomfort, shortness of breath, and fatigue. These symptoms can occur during physical activity or even at rest, depending on the severity of the condition. Symptoms of a stroke can come on suddenly and include numbness or weakness in the face, arm, or leg, especially on one side of the body. Other symptoms are confusion, trouble speaking or understanding speech, difficulty seeing in one or both eyes, and problems walking like dizziness, or unsteady gait. Recognizing these symptoms and immediate hospitalization and medical treatment is crucial in reducing the impact of a stroke.

Occasionally the heart muscle can become very weak and lead to enlargement of the heart size and cause heart failure. This condition is called *Diabetic Cardiomyopathy*.

Prevention and Management

Lifestyle changes are the mainstay in the prevention of CVD in diabetes. Eating a healthy diet that is low in saturated fats, trans fats, cholesterol, and sodium can help manage blood glucose, blood pressure, and cholesterol levels. (See Chapter 18 on *Nutritional Recipes & Meal Plans*). Regular exercise is necessary to improve heart health. It helps to control blood sugar levels and maintain a healthy weight. Quitting smoking is also essential, as smoking damages blood vessels and increases the risk of heart disease. Medications are often necessary to manage cardiovascular risk factors. These include those to lower blood pressure, Statins are medications given to bring down cholesterol levels, and blood thinners (*Antiplatelet agents*) like aspirin to prevent blood clots. Regular monitoring is crucial in preventing and managing cardiovascular disease. Monitoring blood glucose levels, blood pressure, and blood lipid levels is part of the preventive strategy. Working closely with the physician to maintain these levels within normal ranges can significantly reduce the risk of cardiovascular complications.

Below is a table with the normal ranges of various lipids in the blood of an adult. These ranges are generally accepted as indicators of lipid levels in a healthy adult. Values outside these ranges may indicate an increased risk of cardiovascular disease and may require medical attention and lifestyle changes. **(Table 1)**.

Lipid Type	Normal Range mg/dL	Normal Range (mmol/L)
Total Cholesterol	< 200	< 5.2
LDL Cholesterol	< 100	< 2.6
HDL Cholesterol	40 – 60	1.0 – 1.5
Triglycerides	< 150	< 1.7
Non-HDL Cholesterol	< 130	< 3.4

Table 1: Normal Ranges of Lipids

In patients with a pre-existing heart attack (*Myocardial Infarction*) or other cardiovascular diseases, the target lipid levels are often more stringent to reduce the risk of subsequent cardiovascular events. These are given in the table below. These targets are based on guidelines from organizations such as the American Heart Association (AHA) and the American College of Cardiology (ACC). They emphasize the importance of more aggressive lipid-lowering therapy in patients with a history of cardiovascular events to prevent future incidents.

This is always done on the advice of a healthcare professional.
[**Table 2**].

Lipid Type	Target Range Mg/dL	Target Range Mmol/L
Total Cholesterol	150 - 180	3.9 – 4.7
LDL Cholesterol	< 70	< 1.8
HDL Cholesterol	40 – 60	1.0 – 1.5
Triglycerides	< 150	< 1.7
Non-HDL Cholesterol	< 100	< 2.6

Table 2: Lipid Range in Cardiac patients.

DIABETIC NEUROPATHY

Diabetic neuropathy is the nerve damage that occurs in diabetics. It is seen that over 60% of patients with diabetes have some form of neuropathy. There are several types of diabetic neuropathy namely, *Peripheral neuropathy*, *Autonomic neuropathy*, *Proximal neuropathy*, and *Focal neuropathy*. Each type affects different parts of the body in various ways. Neuropathy is quite common in diabetics and can significantly impact their quality of life. Nerve damage leads to pain, discomfort, and other serious health issues, making daily activities more challenging and often disabling. Neuropathy is more common in smokers, tall individuals and those who consume excess alcohol. It tends to occur in those with long standing diabetes and those over 40.

Peripheral Neuropathy

Peripheral neuropathy is the most common type of diabetic neuropathy. *Peripheral* indicates that it is away from the body. Hence it primarily affects the feet and legs, and occasionally the hands and arms.

Symptoms are tingling, numbness, burning sensations, or sharp pin-like pricking pain in these areas. This can lead to severe complications, such as foot ulcers and infections, which can result from the loss of sensation and unnoticed injuries in the feet. The patient fails to notice small cracks or injuries in the sole of the feet, and these may fester to form ulcers. In extreme cases, untreated infections and ulcers can lead to amputations, emphasizing the importance of regular foot care and monitoring in these patients.

Severe neuropathy can lead to a condition called *Neuroarthropathy* where the sensation in the joints is reduced or lost and the patient does not feel joint pain when the joints are injured. This can ultimately lead to deformation of the joints. This can affect the lower limb joints like the knee and ankle. When the knee joint is thus progressively involved causing destruction of the bone and soft tissues of the knee, it is called Charcot's knee as it was described by Jean Martin Charcot in 1868.

Pain and loss of muscle strength in the upper leg and thigh may occur. This is called *Diabetic Amyotrophy*. Sometimes the nerve roots that come out of the spinal cord are affected and these can cause a girdle like pain around the chest or abdomen. This is called *Diabetic Radiculopathy*. Neuropathy affecting the eye muscles can cause squint and drooping of the eyelids.

The doctor tests for neuropathy by testing the vibration sensation with a tuning fork, touch sensation and temperature sensation in the limbs.

Autonomic Neuropathy

Diabetic autonomic neuropathy (**DAN**) affects various autonomic nerve functions, leading to a range of complications. The autonomic nervous system (**ANS**) controls many involuntary body functions, and damage to these nerves can impact multiple systems.

Cardiovascular System

The normal variation of heart rate seen in normal individuals is reduced in DAN leading to an increased and fixed heart rate. A drop in blood pressure (*Hypotension*) upon standing can cause dizziness and fainting.

Gastrointestinal System

Delayed stomach emptying, leading to nausea, vomiting, bloating, and loss of appetite is often seen. Irregular bowel movements causing constipation or sudden, urgent diarrhea may occur in some patients. Difficulty in swallowing due to reduced motility of the food pipe (*Esophagus*) may occur.

Genitourinary System

Difficulty in emptying the bladder completely, leading to urinary retention and infections are seen in some patients, both males and females. Sexual Dysfunction in the form of impotence (*Erectile dysfunction* or ***ED***) may occur in men and reduced vaginal lubrication due to dryness of the vagina in women, causing pain during sexual intercourse. Women also tend to develop fungal infections of the vagina.

Male diabetics develop ED 10-15 years earlier than non-diabetics. It is directly proportional to the number of years the patient has been diabetic. The use of alcohol and tobacco can further aggravate the condition. It has been reported that after the age of seventy, 95% of diabetic males have ED.

Sweating Abnormalities like reduced or excessive sweating may be observed and this may affect temperature regulation. In some patients, abnormal response of the pupils to light, affecting vision, especially in low light conditions may be seen. Reduced ability to recognize low blood sugar levels may occur as they may not develop symptoms like sweating or shakiness. This can increase the risk of severe unrecognized hypoglycemia in such patients.

Diabetic autonomic neuropathy can significantly impact quality of life and requires careful management to address these varied symptoms. Treatment typically focuses on managing the symptoms and strict blood glucose control to prevent further nerve damage.

Mechanisms

Prolonged high blood glucose levels can cause damage to the nerves and the blood vessels that supply them. When blood sugar levels are consistently high, it can interfere with the nerves' ability to transmit signals, thus causing neuropathy. High glucose levels also weaken the walls of the tiny, microscopic blood vessels (*Capillaries*) that supply the nerves with oxygen and nutrients. This lack of blood supply to the nerves further contributes to nerve damage.

Prevention and Management

To prevent and slow the progression of diabetic neuropathy one should maintain a tight control of blood glucose levels. Keeping blood sugar within a target range can help protect the nerves from damage to a great extent. For managing the pain associated with neuropathy, doctors may prescribe medications such as anticonvulsants or antidepressants, which can help alleviate nerve pain. Over-the-counter pain relievers may also be recommended in some cases but may not be beneficial if the neuropathy is severe.

Regular foot care is very important for people with peripheral neuropathy. Daily inspection of the feet for any signs of injury, proper foot hygiene, wearing comfortable shoes that fit well, and getting regular foot exams from a healthcare provider. Early detection and treatment of any foot problems can prevent serious complications.

Understanding the different types of neuropathies and their symptoms is important for diabetics to take proactive steps to manage their condition and maintain their quality of life. Regular medical check-ups, good blood sugar control, and attention to foot care are all essential components of effective neuropathy management.

Focal Neuropathy

Focal neuropathy in diabetes means that only one nerve is affected. This can cause problems in various parts of the body:

<u>Eye Muscles</u>: When focal neuropathy affects the eye muscles, it can lead to double vision. This happens because the eyes are not aligned properly, causing a squint.

<u>Face</u>: If the nerves in the face are involved, it can result in weakness on one side of the face along with inability to close the eyelid, a condition known as *Bell's Palsy*.

<u>Hands</u>: When focal neuropathy affects the nerves in the hand, it often leads to *Carpal Tunnel Syndrome*. This is caused by compression of a nerve called the *Median nerve* at the wrist. The condition causes pain, tingling, and weakness in the hand muscles and fingers.

<u>Feet</u>: If the nerves in the leg are affected, it can cause a condition called *Foot drop*, where lifting the front part of the foot becomes difficult.

<u>**Proximal Neuropathy**</u>

Proximal neuropathy in diabetes involves nerves in the hip, buttocks, or thigh areas. This type of neuropathy has several effects. It causes severe pain in the hip, thigh, buttocks, or legs. The pain can be on one side or both sides of the body. The thigh muscles may become weak, making it hard for the person to stand up from a seated position or to climb stairs. Unlike peripheral neuropathy, which affects small nerves, proximal neuropathy impacts the larger nerves in these areas.

DIABETIC RETINOPATHY

Diabetic retinopathy is a serious eye condition that can develop in people with diabetes. The retina is the light-sensitive layers of nerve tissue lining the back of the eye. It receives images and sends them as electric signals to the brain through the large Optic nerve at the back of the eyeball. Retinopathy is seen equally in males and females and is related to the duration of diabetes. The longer one is diabetic, the more the chances of developing retinopathy. It is one of the leading causes of blindness in adults around the world. There are two main types of diabetic retinopathy: *Non-proliferative* and *Proliferative retinopathy*.

Non-proliferative retinopathy (NPDR) occurs early in the disease and is characterized by the swelling and leaking of blood vessels in the retina. This type does not affect vision and does not worsen over time.

Proliferative retinopathy (PDR) is the more advanced and serious stage and involves the growth of new, abnormal blood vessels in the retina, which can lead to severe vision problems and may cause blindness. It may cause bleeding into the eyeball and detachment of the retina from its anchorage on the wall of the eyeball. Retinopathy tends to occur in diabetics who have high blood pressure and in smokers.

<u>Mechanisms</u>

High blood glucose levels over a long time can damage the small blood vessels in the retina. When these blood vessels are damaged, they leak fluid or bleed, causing swelling in the retina. This causes loss of vision. In advanced stages, the lack of proper blood supply due to blockage of the small vessels in the retina can cause the retina to form new, fragile blood vessels that can break easily and bleed into the eye, further impairing vision. These are grave complications of the disease.

<u>Symptoms</u>

In the early stages of diabetic retinopathy, symptoms may be absent, or the patient might experience mild symptoms such as slightly blurred vision or seeing small spots that appear to drift through the field of vision like insects flying in front of the eye (*Floaters*). As the condition progresses, symptoms might become more severe and significant vision loss, dark or empty areas in the field of vision, and difficulty seeing at night occur. In advanced cases, large areas of vision may be affected, leading to blindness.

<u>Diagnosis</u>

Diabetic retinopathy is often diagnosed by regular eye exams. These exams typically include a dilated retinal examination, where eye drops are used to enlarge the pupils, allowing the doctor to get a better view of the back of the eye (*Retina*).

Other tests, such as Fluorescein Angiography, where a dye is injected into the bloodstream to highlight the blood vessels in the retina, and Optical Coherence Tomography (OCT), which provides detailed images of the retina, are also be used to detect and monitor the progression of the disease.

<u>Prevention and Management</u>

To prevent diabetic retinopathy the blood glucose levels, and blood pressure must be kept under good control. Avoiding smoking is very crucial as smoking can aggravate retinopathy. Regular monitoring of blood sugar levels and maintaining a healthy lifestyle significantly reduce the risk of developing retinopathy. Early detection and treatment of retinopathy are crucial. Treatments for advanced retinopathy include Laser therapy, which seals or shrinks leaking blood vessels. Injections of Anti-VEGF medications can reduce the growth of new blood vessels and decrease swelling in the retina. Surgery, such as *Vitrectomy*, may be needed to remove blood that has leaked into the eye and scar tissue that can cause retinal detachment. Studies have shown that those with retinopathy are twice as likely to have a heart attack.

Thus, by understanding the risks and taking proactive steps to manage their health, people with diabetes can protect their vision and maintain their quality of life. Regular eye check-ups – either yearly or six-monthly, good blood sugar control, and prompt treatment of eye problems are essential in managing diabetic retinopathy effectively.

DIABETIC NEPHROPATHY

Diabetic nephropathy is serious kidney damage that often occurs in people with diabetes. It is one of the leading causes of chronic kidney disease and end-stage renal disease, where the kidneys fail completely and require dialysis or a kidney transplant. Over time, diabetic nephropathy affects the ability of the kidneys to effectively filter waste products from the blood. This leads to a gradual loss of kidney function

Mechanisms

High blood glucose levels persisting for long cause damage to the tiny filtering units in the kidneys which are called *Nephrons*. Each kidney has about one million nephrons. These filters help to remove waste and excess fluids from the blood. When they are damaged the filtration function of the kidney is affected. High blood sugar levels lead to the thickening and scarring of these filters, which results in the kidneys' reduced ability to filter out the unwanted chemicals from the blood.

Symptoms

In the early stages of diabetic nephropathy, symptoms may be absent. One of the first signs can be the presence of a protein called *Albumin* in the urine. Initially, this is present in trace amounts. This condition is known as *Microalbuminuria*. Later the quantity of albumin in urine increases as the disease worsens. Other symptoms may appear as the disease progresses. These are swelling in the legs, ankles, or feet due to fluid retention in the body. In more advanced stages, people experience fatigue, nausea, loss of appetite, and itching. These symptoms are caused by the accumulation of waste products in the body that the kidneys can no longer filter out properly.

Diagnosis

Early changes of Diabetic nephropathy are often detected during regular screening tests. Urine tests are used to check for the presence of albumin (*Microalbuminuria*) which indicates early kidney damage. Blood tests are also performed to assess kidney function by measuring levels of Serum Creatinine and estimating the *Glomerular Filtration Rate* (**eGFR**), which indicates how well the kidneys are filtering the blood.

> *John, a 50-year-old man with a 20-year history of poorly
> controlled diabetes, had recently noticed mild swelling in
> his feet in the evenings and frothy urine. During his
> doctor's visit, John's medical history and symptoms were
> reviewed, followed by a physical examination. Key tests
> included urine analysis for albumin, blood tests for kidney
> function (serum creatinine), and HbA1c to assess long-
> term blood sugar control. His serum creatinine was
> marginally high and his eGFR was reduced. The doctor
> made a diagnosis of Diabetic Nephropathy.*
>
> *To manage his condition, John needed stricter blood sugar
> control, potentially involving medication adjustments and
> the addition of insulin. His blood pressure was better
> controlled with the addition of ACE inhibitors to protect
> his kidneys. Dietary modifications, such as reducing salt
> and protein intake, was recommended. John was put on
> regular follow-up appointments to monitor his kidney
> function, blood pressure, and blood sugar levels. The
> doctor educated him on lifestyle changes and referred him
> to a dietitian for further support. These measures slowed
> the progression of his kidney disease and improved his
> overall health.*

<u>Prevention and Management</u>

Maintaining tight control of blood glucose and blood pressure levels prevents the development of diabetic nephropathy. Keeping these levels within the target range can help reduce the risk of kidney damage. Certain medications such as ACE inhibitors or ARBs are often prescribed to protect kidney function and lower blood pressure. Lifestyle modifications, such as following a healthy diet, exercising regularly, avoiding smoking, and limiting alcohol intake, are also important in managing kidney health. Regular monitoring through blood and urine tests is essential to detect early signs of kidney damage.

By understanding the importance of managing diabetes and taking proactive steps to monitor and protect kidney health, individuals with diabetes can significantly reduce their risk of developing diabetic nephropathy and its associated complications. Regular check-ups with healthcare providers, adherence to prescribed treatments, and healthy lifestyle choices play a crucial role in maintaining kidney function and overall health.

FOOT COMPLICATIONS

People with diabetes are at a high risk for foot problems which include ulcers, infections, occasionally leading to amputations. This increased risk is due to several factors. Nerve damage (*Neuropathy*), poor blood circulation due to disease of the blood vessels caused by atherosclerosis, and a weakened immune system all are causative in the development of diabetic foot problems. Neuropathy can lead to a loss of sensation in the feet, making it difficult to notice injuries or pressure sores. Poor circulation can slow down the healing process, and immune dysfunction can make infections more likely and harder to treat.

<u>Common Issues</u>

Foot ulcers are open sores that can develop from minor injuries, pressure, or friction. These ulcers are more likely to occur in people with diabetes because of their reduced ability to feel pain and pressure due to neuropathy. Risk factors for foot ulcers include poorly fitting footwear, calluses, and foot deformities. Symptoms of foot ulcers include redness, swelling, and drainage of pus from the sore.

Infections in the legs and feet are another common problem for diabetics. Because of their compromised immune systems, they are more susceptible to infections. Even minor cuts or blisters can become seriously infected, leading to complications that may require hospitalization. Signs of infection include increased pain, redness, warmth around the wound, pus, and fever.

Cellulitis is a common bacterial infection that affects the deeper layers of the skin and subcutaneous tissues. This can occur in the legs of diabetics causing redness, swelling, pain, and inflammation in the infected area. If not treated promptly, cellulitis can spread and lead to serious health issues.

<u>Prevention and Management</u>

Regular foot examinations are needed to prevent foot complications. These should preferably be done by a healthcare professional regularly. The patient should check his feet daily at home. A mirror may be used to check the soles of the feet. If he is unable to do it, a caregiver or a relative should help him in inspecting the feet.

- Proper foot care includes keeping the feet clean and moisturized. Feet should be washed with warm water and mild soap. Harsh soaps should be avoided. The spaces between the toes should be dried well after washing. Moisturizer should not be applied between the toes.
- Protecting the feet from heat and cold is essential. Avoid using hot pads on the feet. Avoid excess heat in electric blankets.
- Trimming toenails carefully and cutting the toenails straight and smoothing the edges with Emory paper or board is necessary to avoid injury to the adjacent toe. The nails should not be cut too short. One should be careful to avoid injuring the skin while cutting the nails.

Those with poor vision should seek help from a caregiver.

- Wearing socks and shoes that fit well and protect the feet is important. Prefer cotton socks. Wearing appropriate footwear is crucial to prevent injuries and ulcers to the feet. Leather, canvas or suede shoes are ideal. Do not use plastic or materials that do not 'breathe'. Avoid high heels. Shoes should fit properly, have enough room in the front to avoid pressure points, and provide support and cushioning. Prefer shoes with adjustable laces buckles or Velcro which permits adjusting the pressure on the feet.
- Never attempt to remove corn or calluses oneself.
- Never walk barefoot, especially outdoors. Wear comfortable footwear indoors. Remove shoes every 4 - 5 hours. Always check shoes before wearing them for any pebbles or tears inside.
- Any cuts, blisters, or sores should be treated promptly. Any discoloration noticed in the feet should be brought to the attention of the doctor. Even minor wounds should be cleaned and monitored for signs of infection. If a wound does not heal or shows signs of infection, medical attention should be sought promptly.
- Managing foot complications often requires a team approach. This can include foot doctors (*Podiatrists*) diabetes specialists (*Endocrinologists*), and wound care specialists. Together, they can provide comprehensive care to prevent and treat foot problems in people with diabetes.

Patients with diabetes should be taught how to inspect their feet daily. Good foot hygiene is essential. Patients should be encouraged to seek medical help if they notice any abnormalities, such as wounds that do not heal, signs of infection, or changes in skin color or temperature. Early intervention can prevent minor issues from becoming serious complications.

By understanding the importance of foot care and taking proactive steps, individuals with diabetes can significantly reduce their risk of developing serious foot problems. Regular check-ups with healthcare providers, proper footwear, and good self-care practices are essential for maintaining healthy feet and preventing complications.

SKIN DISEASES

People with diabetes often experience various skin conditions due to high blood sugar levels and poor circulation. Here are some common skin problems associated with diabetes, along with their descriptions:

Infections

Fungal Infections: These are caused by fungi and are common in moist areas like the groin, armpits, and between the toes. Conditions like jock itch (*Tinea cruris*), ringworm (*Tinea corporis*) and athlete's foot (*Tinea pedis*) are examples. Fungal infections can occur in the nails. The nails, especially toenails, can become thick, yellow, and brittle due to fungal infections.

Bacterial Infections: Bacterial infections, such as an infection around the nails (*Paronychia*), can also occur more frequently in people with diabetes. Boils can also occur frequently in diabetes. *Carbuncles* are skin infections caused by the bacteria named staphylococci. It can extend deep in the skin and may exude pus.

Necrobiosis Lipoidica

This condition usually affects the shins and ankles. It appears as patches of reddish-brown skin that can become shiny and cause the skin to become thin.

Xanthelasma

These are small, yellow, flat areas that appear on the eyelids. They are deposits of fat and are more common in people with diabetes.

Alopecia

Hair loss can occur in people with diabetes due to poor blood circulation and hormonal changes.

Insulin Hypertrophy

This happens when fatty tissue accumulates at the site of insulin injections. It can cause lumps and affect the absorption of insulin.

Insulin Lipoatrophy

This condition is characterized by the loss of fat at the injection site, leading to indentations in the skin.

Dry Skin

High blood sugar levels can cause the skin to become dry and itchy. Poor circulation can also reduce the skin's ability to heal, leading to cracks and infections.

Intertrigo

This is an inflammation caused by skin-to-skin friction, often occurring in warm, moist areas like the groin, under the breasts in women, and between the toes.

Acanthosis Nigricans

This condition causes velvety, dark plaques to develop on the neck, back, and armpits. It is often associated with insulin resistance.

Diabetic Dermopathy

Often referred to as 'shin spots,' this condition appears as light brown, scaly patches on the front of the legs.

Diabetic Thick Skin

After living with diabetes for over 10 years, some people may develop thick, waxy skin, especially on the fingers and toes.

Bullosis Diabeticorum

This condition, also known as diabetic blisters, causes spontaneous blisters to appear on the skin of the fingers, hands, toes, and feet. They are painless and look like burns.

Eruptive Xanthomatosis

This condition is characterized by the sudden appearance of yellow, pea-like bumps on the skin. It is often associated with high blood fats and poor blood sugar control.

Managing blood sugar levels effectively can help reduce the risk of developing these skin conditions. Additionally, proper skin care, including moisturizing, good hygiene, and prompt treatment of cuts and infections, is crucial for maintaining healthy skin.

GUM DISEASE

People with diabetes are more prone to gum disease due to high blood sugar levels, which create an environment in the mouth that encourages bacteria to thrive. When blood sugar levels are high, sugar levels in the mouth also increase. This excess sugar provides food for harmful bacteria, which multiply more rapidly. These bacteria then form a sticky film called *plaque* on the teeth and gums. Plaque build-up on the teeth and gums can lead to infections. The body's response to this infection causes the gums to become inflamed. This inflammation of the gums is known as *Gingivitis*. Gingivitis is the early stage of gum disease. It causes the gums to become red, swollen, and more likely to bleed, especially during brushing or flossing. If gingivitis is not treated, it can progress to a more severe form of gum disease called *Periodontitis*.

Periodontitis occurs when the inflammation spreads below the gum line, causing the gums to pull away from the teeth. This creates pockets that can lodge food particles and become infected. Over time, the bone and tissues supporting the teeth can be destroyed, leading to loosening of teeth and tooth loss.

Maintaining proper dental hygiene is crucial for preventing gum disease. This includes brushing teeth at least twice a day, flossing daily, and using an antibacterial mouthwash. Managing blood sugar levels effectively can also help reduce the risk of gum disease. People with diabetes should visit their dentist at least twice a year for professional cleaning and checkups. Regular dental visits can help detect early signs of gum disease and prevent its progression. In addition to regular dental care, people with diabetes should avoid smoking, as it can further increase the risk of gum disease. Eating a balanced diet and staying hydrated are also important for maintaining oral health.

If gum disease is left untreated, it can lead to serious complications. These include chronic bad breath, pain while chewing, and ultimately, loss of teeth. Gum disease can also have a negative impact on overall health, potentially leading to other complications in people with diabetes.

OTHER HEALTH ASSOCIATIONS IN PATIENTS WITH DIABETES

People with diabetes often face additional health challenges beyond blood sugar control. Some significant associations that have been observed are:

High Risk of Cancer

Individuals with diabetes have a higher risk of dying from certain types of cancer, including breast cancer, liver cancer, and colon cancer. This increased risk is linked to high blood sugar levels and insulin resistance, which can promote cancer cell growth.

Arthritis and Bone Fractures

There is a high incidence of arthritis among people with diabetes. Joint pain and stiffness can be more pronounced, making movement difficult. Additionally, people with diabetes are more prone to bone fractures. Poor bone health and complications from nerve damage increase the risk of falls and subsequent fractures.

Psoriasis

Psoriasis, a chronic skin condition that causes red, scaly patches, is more common in individuals with diabetes. The exact connection is not entirely understood, but it is believed that inflammation and immune system changes play a role.

<u>Higher Incidence of Falls in Elderly Diabetics</u>

Elderly people with diabetes are at a higher risk of falling. This is due to a combination of factors including poor vision, nerve damage, and muscle weakness. Falls can lead to serious injuries, such as hip fractures, which can significantly impact quality of life.

<u>Increased Risk of Cognitive Impairment</u>

Diabetes is associated with an increased risk of cognitive impairment and dementia. High blood sugar levels over time can damage blood vessels in the brain, leading to memory problems and reduced cognitive function. Managing blood sugar levels is crucial to help maintain brain health.

<u>Sleep Apnea</u>

Sleep apnea is more common in individuals with diabetes especially when they are obese. This condition causes breathing to stop and start repeatedly during sleep, leading to poor sleep quality and increased risk of cardiovascular problems.

Being aware of these associations helps individuals with diabetes and their caregivers take proactive steps to manage these risks. This includes regular check-ups, maintaining a healthy lifestyle, and adhering to prescribed treatments to help mitigate these additional health challenges.

Chapter 9 – BLOOD GLUCOSE MONITORING

This chapter focuses on the critical aspect of blood glucose monitoring in diabetes management. Regular monitoring of blood sugar levels is essential for managing diabetes effectively and preventing complications. We will discuss the importance of keeping track of blood glucose levels, which helps in making informed decisions about diet, exercise, and medications. Different types of devices used for monitoring, such as traditional blood glucose meters and continuous glucose monitors (CGMs), will be explored. You will learn about the target blood sugar levels to aim for, and the Importance of individualized targets set by your healthcare provider. Additionally, how to interpret the results from these devices, helping you understand what your readings mean and how to respond appropriately, will be explained. By educating yourself on proper blood glucose monitoring, you can take control of your diabetes and maintain a healthier lifestyle.

Importance of Blood Glucose Monitoring

Regular monitoring of blood glucose is important in the effective management of diabetes. This helps patients understand how different factors like food, exercise, and medications affect their blood sugar. For instance, they can see how a particular meal raises their blood sugar or how a workout lowers it. This helps them to make decisions about what to eat, how much to exercise, and when to take medications. It gives them a clear picture of how the body responds to various daily activities, aiding better overall control of diabetes.

Preventing Complications

Regular monitoring of blood glucose levels plays a key role in preventing diabetic complications. Acute complications like low blood sugar (*hypoglycemia*) and high blood sugar (*hyperglycemia*) can thus be avoided. Additionally, regular monitoring helps the patient prevent long-term complications such as cardiovascular disease, nerve damage (*neuropathy*), and eye problems (*retinopathy*) early and take appropriate action. By detecting these issues early, they can be managed more effectively.

Personalized Diabetes Management

Each person's body reacts differently to food, physical activity, and medications. Monitoring blood sugar levels helps them to adjust their diet, exercise routine, and medication regimen to their specific needs. This personalized approach helps in achieving better blood sugar control. Doctors can use the data from monitoring to make appropriate changes to treatment plans, ensuring effective management of diabetes.

<u>Improving Quality of Life</u>

The quality of life of the person significantly improves when blood glucose is regularly monitored. When blood sugar levels are well-managed, people generally feel healthier and more energetic. They can engage in daily activities with less worry about sudden fluctuations in blood sugar. This improved control reduces their anxiety regarding diabetes management and increases their confidence in handling the condition. Knowing that their blood sugar is stable allows individuals to live more comfortably and with greater peace of mind, enhancing their overall well-being.

Types of Monitoring Devices

Some of the currently used devices for monitoring blood glucose are discussed below.

<u>Traditional Blood Glucose Meters</u>

These devices are used to measure blood glucose levels by analyzing a small drop of blood, usually taken from the fingertip. These blood glucose meters are widely used and are considered reliable for checking blood sugar levels at specific times during the day. The key components of these devices include test strips in which the blood sample is introduced; lancets, which are small needles used to prick the skin and obtain the blood drop; and the meter itself, which reads the test strip and displays the blood glucose level digitally. Before using the blood glucose meter, the patient should wash his hands and dry them thoroughly. A test strip is inserted into the meter, using a lancet the fingertip is pricked to get a drop of blood which is then placed on the test strip. The reading on the meter gives the blood glucose level. These devices have a memory function which stores the various readings and hence are useful while going to the physician for checkup. They can be downloaded onto a computer.

Continuous Glucose Monitors (CGMs)

Continuous Glucose Monitors (CGMs) are more advanced devices that offer real-time glucose readings round the clock. These monitors are very useful as they continuously track glucose levels, providing a comprehensive picture of how blood sugar changes throughout the day and night. The components of a CGM are a small sensor that is inserted under the skin, typically on the abdomen or arm; a transmitter that sends glucose data from the sensor to a display device which is kept outside; and a receiver or display device, such as a smartphone or a dedicated monitor, where the glucose readings are seen. CGMs measure glucose levels in the fluid between the cells (*interstitial fluid*) and not from blood. This continuous monitoring allows for the detection of trends and patterns, helping individuals make more informed decisions about their diet, activity, and medication. CGMs are very useful devices for those who need to closely monitor their glucose levels frequently and manage their diabetes more effectively.

Flash Glucose Monitoring Systems

Flash Glucose Monitoring Systems are another type of glucose monitoring technology helping to check the glucose levels quickly and easily. These systems consist of a small sensor that is worn on the skin, typically on the upper arm, and a scanning device. To get a glucose reading, users simply scan the sensor with the scanning device, which displays the current glucose level. Unlike CGMs, flash glucose monitors do not provide continuous real-time readings but offer a convenient method of checking glucose levels without the need to draw blood. Flash glucose monitors are particularly appealing for their ease of use and the ability to scan as often as needed to get a snapshot of glucose levels.

<u>Advanced Features and Integration</u>

Modern glucose monitoring devices come with a variety of advanced features that have improved their functionality and user experience. Many of these advanced devices can integrate with smartphones and other smart devices through apps and software. This allows detailed data analysis and tracking of blood glucose levels. These apps can help users understand their glucose patterns, set goals, and make better decisions about their diabetes management. Some devices also include alerts and alarms that notify users when their glucose levels are too high or too low, providing an extra layer of safety and helping to prevent emergencies. Many monitoring systems also offer data sharing capabilities, which allow users to share their glucose data with their physicians, caregivers, and family members. This sharing can facilitate better communication and support in managing diabetes, ensuring that everyone involved is informed and can contribute to effective diabetes care.

Using these various devices, patients with diabetes can manage their blood sugar levels more effectively. Whether using traditional blood glucose meters, continuous glucose monitors, flash glucose monitoring systems, or benefiting from advanced features and integration, regular monitoring is the most important part of managing diabetes.

Frequency and Targets for Monitoring

How frequently should one monitor blood glucose levels in diabetes to maintain good health is important in management?

<u>Recommended Monitoring Frequency</u>

<u>Type 1 Diabetes</u>: For people with T1DM, frequent monitoring throughout the day is needed to ensure that the

blood glucose levels stay within a safe range. This hence needs blood glucose levels to be checked multiple times daily - before and after meals, before bedtime, and sometimes during the night. The exact frequency can vary based on individual treatment plans and needs based on the advice of the physician, but the goal is to maintain good control over blood sugar levels to prevent extreme fluctuations.

Type 2 Diabetes: For those with T2DM, the frequency of monitoring can vary widely depending on the treatment regimen and on the advice of the treating physician. Some patients might only need to check their blood sugar levels a few times a week if their diabetes is well-controlled with diet and oral medications. Those on insulin or more complex treatment plans, might need to monitor daily or multiple times a day. The healthcare provider will advise depending on the individual's specific circumstances and treatment goals.

Gestational Diabetes: During pregnancy, women with GDM need to monitor their blood glucose levels carefully to protect the health of the mother and baby. Often checking blood sugar levels several times a day may be needed. This helps ensure that glucose levels remain stable and within a healthy range throughout the pregnancy. The doctor's advice is important.

Target Blood Glucose Ranges

General Targets for Non-Pregnant Adults with Diabetes: For adults with diabetes who are not pregnant, there are generally recommended target ranges for blood glucose levels.

Fasting blood glucose should be between **80-130 mg/dL (4.4-7.2 mmol/L)**.

After food, (*postprandial glucose*), the goal is to keep blood sugar below **180 mg/dL (10.0 mmol/L)** one to two hours after the start of a meal. These targets help in managing diabetes effectively and preventing complications.

Individualized Targets: It is important to note that blood glucose targets can be adjusted based on individual factors such as age, other associated health conditions (*Comorbidities*), and personal health goals. For example, older adults or those with significant health issues might have slightly higher targets to avoid the risks associated with very low blood sugar levels. The healthcare provider will work with the individual to set personalized targets that are safe and achievable.

Special Considerations

More frequent monitoring or adjustments are required in certain special situations to achieve blood glucose targets. For example, during periods of illness, stress, or significant changes in daily routine (like travel or changes in physical activity), blood sugar levels can fluctuate more than usual. In such cases, it is important to monitor blood glucose more frequently to detect and manage any significant changes.

Frequent monitoring is also needed when medications are changed, adjusted or new medications started. This helps to assess how the new treatment is affecting blood sugar levels and to make appropriate adjustments in dosage. Regular communication with the doctor during these times is necessary to ensure that the blood glucose levels remain stable and within the target range.

Interpreting Results

Understanding Glucose Patterns

Monitoring blood glucose levels over time is important in the effective management of diabetes. Consistent recording of blood sugar readings can identify patterns and trends that provide insights into how the body responds to different foods, activities, and medications. For example, one might notice that blood sugar tends to spike after eating a certain meal or drop after specific physical activities. Recognizing these patterns one makes decisions about the diet, exercise, and medication to maintain stable blood sugar levels.

It is important to focus on overall trends rather than individual readings. One should not be overly concerned about a single low reading if there are no symptoms. But if the readings are consistently high or low it indicates that adjustments will be needed in the diabetes management plan. This approach allows for more accurate and effective management of diabetes.

Recognizing Hypoglycemia

Hypoglycemia occurs when the blood sugar level drops below 70 mg/dL, which can be dangerous if not treated promptly. Hypoglycemia is recognized by symptoms such as shakiness, sweating, confusion, and dizziness. If one experiences symptoms of low blood sugar, immediate action is needed. Fast-acting carbohydrates like glucose tablets, juice, or candy to raise the blood sugar quickly should be taken. After consuming these, blood sugar levels should be rechecked to ensure they are back in the safe range. If symptoms persist or the blood sugar does not improve, medical advice should be sought promptly.

Recognizing Hyperglycemia

Hyperglycemia refers to high blood sugar levels, which can also lead to serious complications if not managed properly. One should identify blood sugar readings that are very high. Symptoms are excessive thirst, frequent urination, fatigue, and blurred vision. To manage high blood sugar, one needs to adjust the medication, make dietary changes, or increase one's intake of fluids. Monitoring one's diet strictly to avoid foods high in sugar and carbs, and staying hydrated, helps manage hyperglycemia. If high blood sugar levels persist, the doctor should be consulted for further guidance.

<u>Using Data for Long-Term Management</u>

Consistently recording and analyzing one's blood glucose readings helps the patient, and the doctor make decisions about long-term diabetes management. This helps to plan a better control of the patient's blood sugar levels. These records can show how effective the current treatment plan is and help identify any necessary changes. Working closely with the doctor to review this data helps to manage the disease better.

<u>Psychological Aspects</u>

Some patients find regularly monitoring and interpreting blood glucose levels stressful and emotionally challenging. It is normal to feel anxious or overwhelmed by the responsibility of managing one's diabetes. Hence, developing strategies to cope with this stress becomes important. Seeking support from family and friends, joining a diabetes support group, or working with a mental health professional may be needed in some patients. By addressing the emotional impact of diabetes management, one can reduce stress and improve overall well-being.

Chapter 10 - LIFESTYLE MANAGEMENT

This chapter explains in brief the critical role of lifestyle management in controlling diabetes. Effective diabetes management goes beyond medications; it encompasses a comprehensive approach involving diet, exercise, and other lifestyle changes. We will explore the importance of a balanced diet, focusing on nutritional guidelines that can help maintain stable blood glucose levels. You will learn about the significance of regular physical activity and how different types of exercise can benefit your overall health and diabetes control. Other relevant lifestyle factors, such as stress management and adequate sleep, which are essential in maintaining optimal health, will also be discussed. The chapter emphasizes patient education, providing practical tips and strategies to help you make informed choices and take proactive steps in managing your diabetes. By adopting a healthy lifestyle, you can significantly improve your quality of life and reduce the risk of diabetes-related complications. More detailed information about the individual components are available in other chapters.

Importance of Diet and Nutrition

Role in Diabetes Management

Diet and nutrition are important because what you eat directly affects your blood sugar levels. When foods high in carbohydrates are consumed the blood sugar levels rise. Managing what one eats and when helps keep these levels stable, preventing highs and lows. A balanced diet, rich in essential nutrients and low in unhealthy fats and sugars, helps manage diabetes effectively. Eating a wide variety of foods ensures that one gets the necessary vitamins and minerals that are needed for good health and preventing complications related to diabetes.

Weight Management

A healthy weight is essential for diabetics as it directly affects how well the body responds to insulin. Weight management improves insulin sensitivity thereby making blood sugar control easier. Achieving and maintaining a healthy weight through a balanced diet and regular physical activity can significantly improve diabetes management. In addition, it helps to reduce the risk of heart disease, improves blood pressure, and enhances overall well-being, making it an important aspect diabetes care.

Prevention of Complications

Adhering to a proper diet helps prevent or delay the onset of complications of diabetes, such as heart disease, nerve damage (*neuropathy*), and kidney disease (*nephropathy*). Foods that are low in sugar and unhealthy fats, and high in fiber, protect the organs and keep the blood vessels healthy. Certain nutrients, like antioxidants found in fruits and vegetables, are important to support overall health and reduce the risk of diabetes-related complications. Omega-3 fatty acids, found in fish and flaxseeds, are beneficial for heart health, while whole grains and legumes provide fiber that helps regulate blood sugar levels. [See Chapter 18 on *Nutritional Recipes and Meal Plans*].

<u>Quality of Life</u>

A healthy diet affects one's energy levels, mood, and overall sense of well-being. Eating nutritious meals regularly can help one feel more energetic and less fatigued, making it easier to manage daily activities and exercise. Proper nutrition also helps in supporting the mental health of diabetics. Enjoying a variety of healthy foods can also make mealtimes more enjoyable and less restrictive.

Dietary Guidelines for Diabetes

Let us briefly discuss regarding some dietary guidelines for diabetic patients. These will be discussed in more detail later. [See Chapter 18 on *Nutritional Recipes and Meal Plans*].

Carbohydrate Counting

<u>What is Carbohydrate Counting?</u>

Carbohydrate counting is the method used to manage blood glucose levels by tracking the amount of carbohydrates one eats. Carbohydrates are the main component of food that affects blood sugar levels, hence monitoring their intake helps keep these levels within a target range. Understanding how different foods impact one's blood sugar helps in making informed dietary choices.

<u>How to Count Carbohydrates?</u>

Counting carbohydrates involves knowing how many grams of carbs are present in the foods that one eats. Food labels often list the carbohydrate content. A measuring cup or a food scale may be used to ensure accurate portion sizes. Many resources, such as carbohydrate counting books, mobile apps, and online databases, can help a diabetic determine the carb content of foods without labels, like fruits, vegetables and grains. Keeping a food diary also helps track one's intake.

<u>Balancing Carbohydrates with Insulin</u>

In patients on insulin therapy, balancing carbohydrate intake with insulin doses is very important. Eating a consistent amount of carbohydrates at each meal helps predict how much insulin one needs to manage the blood sugar levels. It is important to adjust one's carbohydrate intake and insulin doses during activities that affect blood sugar, such as exercise, illness, or changes in daily routine. Consulting with one's doctor can help develop a personalized plan for managing these adjustments.

<u>Benefits of Carbohydrate Counting</u>

Carbohydrate counting leads to better blood glucose control, allowing more flexibility in food choices and meal planning. It empowers the patient to enjoy a wider variety of foods – even sweets, while still managing diabetes effectively. By understanding the impact of different foods on blood sugar levels, one can make more informed choices and reduce the risk of blood sugar highs and lows. This information can lead to a more balanced and satisfying diet, improving overall health and well-being.

Glycemic Index

<u>What is the Glycemic Index (**GI**)?</u>

The *Glycemic Index* is a tool to measure how quickly foods containing carbohydrates raise blood glucose levels after being consumed. Foods are ranked on a scale from 0 to 100, with pure glucose scoring 100. This ranking helps understand how different foods affect blood sugar.

Foods with a high GI (70 and above) cause rapid rise in blood sugar levels, while medium GI foods (56-69) cause moderate increases and low GI foods (55 and below) result in slower, more gradual rises in blood sugar. This knowledge is important for managing diabetes to maintain steady blood sugar levels.

<u>How to Use the Glycemic Index</u>

Incorporating low and medium GI foods into one's diet can be beneficial in managing diabetes. Examples of low GI foods include most fruits, vegetables, legumes, and whole grains. These foods release glucose more slowly while being digested, helping to keep blood sugar levels stable. High GI foods, such as white bread, sugary cereals, white rice, refined wheat flour (*Maida*) and baked goods, can cause quick spikes in blood sugar. As far as possible, they should be replaced by healthier options. For instance, choosing whole grain bread instead of white bread, and opting for brown rice over white rice or whole wheat instead of refined wheat flour helps. Small changes like these can make a significant difference.

<u>Benefits of a Low GI Diet</u>

A low GI diet can help maintain more stable blood glucose levels. This results in fewer sharp rises and falls. Stable blood sugar levels can also lead to more consistent energy levels throughout the day. Over the long term, a low GI diet can help weight management because it helps control hunger and reduces the chances of overeating. It can also improve cardiovascular health by lowering cholesterol levels and reducing the risk of heart disease.

<u>Combining GI with Other Dietary Approaches</u>

While the glycemic index is a useful tool, it is important to combine it with other dietary strategies for the best results. For example carbohydrate counting and low glycemic index foods together provide a better approach to managing blood sugar levels. This combination ensures that one not only chooses the right *types* of carbohydrates but also monitors the *quantity* consumed.

Portion sizes and overall nutritional balance are also important while eating. Eating a balanced diet that includes a variety of nutrients from different food groups that support overall health. For instance, adding proteins and healthy fats to meals can slow the absorption of carbohydrates, further helping to stabilize blood sugar levels. Using all these approaches a well-rounded diet plan can be created to make the management of diabetes easier.

Meal Planning

Creating a Balanced Meal Plan

A balanced meal plan for diabetes should include all the key nutrients - carbohydrates, proteins, fats, fiber, and essential vitamins and minerals. Carbohydrates are the main source of energy and should be chosen carefully to maintain stable blood sugar levels. Proteins help build and repair tissues, while healthy fats support cell function and hormone production. Fiber is essential for digestive health and helps to slow down the absorption of sugars, thereby preventing spikes in blood glucose levels. Meals should be eaten at regular times each day and one must be mindful of portion sizes. Regular meal timing helps to maintain consistent and smooth blood sugar levels, while portion control helps to control the quantity of carbs consumed.

Planning Meals and Snacks

When planning meals and snacks, it is essential to consider how different foods affect one's blood sugar. Aiming to include a mix of low GI carbohydrates, lean proteins, and healthy fats in each meal is important to help keep blood glucose levels stable. For instance, a balanced breakfast might include whole grain toast with avocado and a boiled egg, while a healthy snack could be a small handful of nuts, or a piece of fruit paired with a piece of cheese. Examples of balanced meals could include grilled chicken with a quinoa salad and steamed vegetables, or a vegetarian option like a lentil stew with a side of brown rice and a green salad. Healthy snacks might include Greek yogurt with a sprinkle of chia seeds, or carrot sticks with hummus. These combinations provide the necessary nutrients while helping to maintain steady blood sugar levels. [See Chapter 18 on *Nutritional Recipes & Meal Plans*].

<u>Adapting Meal Plans to Individual Needs</u>

It is important to tailor meal plans to fit individual preferences, lifestyles, and cultural practices. There is no 'one size fits all' option in diabetic diet. This ensures that the meal plan is enjoyable and sustainable in the long term. For example, if you have a busy schedule, you might prefer quick and easy meals that can be prepared in advance. If you follow a specific cultural diet like a South Indian Vegetarian diet, you can incorporate traditional foods that are suitable for diabetes management. Flexibility and variety are key to maintaining long-term adherence to any meal plan. It is important to have a range of meal options to choose from so that one does not get bored with one's diet. Including different foods from all food groups ensures that the diabetic gets a variety of nutrients and helps to keep meals interesting and enjoyable.

<u>Working with a Dietitian</u>

Getting help from a registered dietitian can be a valuable resource in creating and adjusting meal plans for diabetes management. Dietitians are trained to understand the nutritional needs of individuals with diabetes and can provide personalized advice based on your health goals, cultural preferences, and lifestyle.

Emily, a 26-year-old college student, discovered she had a BMI of 29 during a routine checkup. Given her family history—her father and maternal uncle both had diabetes—her doctor advised her on the importance of taking proactive steps to manage her weight and reduce her risk of developing diabetes.

The doctor emphasized the significance of a healthy diet, recommending Emily to focus on whole foods such as vegetables, fruits, whole grains, and lean proteins while reducing her intake of processed foods, sugary snacks, and beverages. Portion control and balanced meals were crucial for her weight management. In addition to dietary changes, the doctor advised Emily to increase her physical activity. Engaging in at least 150 minutes of moderate aerobic exercise per week, such as brisk walking, swimming, or cycling, was recommended. Incorporating strength training exercises twice a week was advised to improve her overall fitness and metabolism. The doctor also suggested regular monitoring of her blood sugar levels, given her family history, and scheduling follow-up appointments to track her progress. Emily was encouraged to maintain a healthy weight, aiming for gradual weight loss if needed, as even a modest reduction in weight could significantly decrease her risk of diabetes.

Emily took up 45 minutes of swimming daily and followed a strict diet prescribed by her dietitian. By adopting these lifestyle changes, Emily effectively managed her weight and hopes to prevent or delay the onset of diabetes.

Diets vary from person to person and from region to region. Professional guidance from a dietitian helps one make informed choices about diet, ensuring that one gets the right balance of nutrients. Dietitians can also help one navigate challenges such as eating out, managing special occasions, or dealing with dietary restrictions. Their support can make a significant difference in successfully managing diabetes through diet.

Physical Activity and Exercise

A brief discussion on the importance of exercise is given here. More details may be found in chapter 17 on *Exercise & Physical Activity Plans*.

<u>Role of Exercise in Diabetes Management</u>

Regular physical activity is essential for people with diabetes. Exercise helps the body use insulin more effectively, lower blood sugar levels and maintain a healthy weight. It also reduces the risk of heart disease and other complications. Besides the physical benefits, exercise also has a positive impact on mental health. It helps to reduce stress, anxiety, and depression, leading to an improved mood and a better sense of well-being. Regular physical activity can also boost energy levels and promote better sleep.

<u>Recommended Exercise Guidelines</u>

Health experts recommend that individuals with diabetes should aim for at least 150 minutes of moderate-intensity aerobic activity each week. This can include activities like brisk walking, cycling, or swimming. In addition to aerobic exercise, it is important to include muscle-strengthening activities, such as lifting weights, using Resistance Bands or doing bodyweight exercises, on two or more days per week. Consistency is very important when it comes to exercise. It is important to start slowly and gradually increase the intensity and duration of your workouts. Such a 'warm up' and 'cool down' approach helps to prevent injuries and ensures that exercise becomes a sustainable part of one's routine.

<u>Monitoring Blood Glucose During Exercise</u>

Monitoring blood sugar levels is important before, during, and after exercise. This helps to understand how physical activity affects blood glucose levels and to ensure they remain within a safe range. Checking one's blood sugar before starting exercise can help one determine if a snack is needed to prevent low blood sugar while exercising. Adjusting one's exercise routine based on blood glucose readings is crucial. For instance, if a person's blood sugar is too low before exercising, he should eat a small snack. If it is too high, he might need to wait until it comes down to a safer level before starting the workout.

<u>Safety Considerations</u>

Staying hydrated during exercising is essential, as dehydration can affect blood sugar levels. It is also important to wear appropriate footwear to prevent foot injuries, especially for those with diabetes-related complications like neuropathy. It is also preferable to wear light, loose clothing like cotton clothes. Taking adequate precautions is vital for individuals with diabetes-related complications such as nerve damage (*neuropathy*) or cardiovascular disease. Consulting with one's doctor is essential to ensure that the exercise plan is safe and appropriate for the patient.

Types of Exercise

<u>Aerobic Exercise</u>

Aerobic exercises are activities that increase one's heart rate and make one breathe harder. Examples include walking, jogging, swimming, and cycling. These activities help improve cardiovascular health, which is particularly important for people with diabetes. Regular aerobic exercise can also lead to better blood glucose control and enhance overall fitness levels.

Resistance Training

Resistance training involves exercises that improve muscle strength and endurance. This includes weightlifting, bodyweight exercises like push-ups and squats, or using resistance bands. Building muscle through resistance training improves insulin sensitivity, making it easier for the body to manage blood sugar levels. It also helps improve body composition by increasing muscle mass and reducing body fat.

Flexibility and Balance Exercises

Flexibility and balance exercises are activities that help improve the range of motion and stability of the body. Examples include yoga, stretching, and tai chi. These exercises can enhance flexibility, improve balance, and reduce the risk of falls, which is particularly beneficial for older adults and those with diabetes-related complications.

Integrating Different Types of Exercise

A well-rounded exercise program including a mix of aerobic, resistance, and flexibility training should be regularly practiced. This approach ensures that one reaps the benefits of each type of exercise and maintains a balanced fitness routine. For instance, one might go for a brisk walk on some days, lift weights on others, and practice yoga to improve flexibility and balance.

Incorporating physical activity into one's daily routine can be enjoyable and sustainable. Simple changes like taking the stairs instead of the elevator, walking or cycling to nearby places, playing with your children, gardening or even dancing to your favorite music can make a big difference. Finding activities one enjoys will help a person stay motivated and make exercise a regular part of one's life.

Additional Aspects of Lifestyle

In managing diabetes, lifestyle changes go beyond diet and exercise. Here are some additional crucial aspects that a patient with diabetes should focus on:

Stress Management

Chronic stress can raise blood sugar levels and make diabetes management more challenging. It is important for patients to adopt stress-reducing techniques like mindfulness meditation, deep breathing exercises, and engaging in hobbies that promote relaxation. Regular breaks and ensuring a good work-life balance can also help keep stress levels in check.

Sleep Quality

Poor sleep can negatively impact blood sugar levels and overall health. Patients should aim for 7-9 hours of quality sleep each night. Establishing a regular sleep schedule, creating a restful environment, and avoiding stimulants like caffeine before bedtime can improve sleep. Alcohol can also disrupt one's sleep. If sleep problems persist, consulting a healthcare provider is important to rule out conditions like sleep apnea, which is common in people with diabetes.

Smoking Cessation and Alcohol Moderation

Smoking can increase the risk of diabetes complications, particularly cardiovascular issues. Quitting smoking is essential for reducing these risks. Similarly, alcohol should be consumed in moderation, as it can affect blood sugar levels and interact with diabetes medications. Patients should follow their healthcare provider's guidelines on safe alcohol consumption.

By following these guidelines and incorporating a variety of exercises into one's routine, a diabetic can effectively manage his blood sugar and improve your overall health. Regular physical activity is a powerful tool in maintaining stable blood sugar levels, enhancing well-being, and preventing complications. The reader is advised to read this chapter in conjunction with the chapter on *Exercise and Physical Activity Plans*.

Chapter 11 - DIABETES IN SPECIAL POPULATIONS

Diabetes affects people of all ages and backgrounds, but certain groups require special attention and care. In this chapter, we will explore the unique challenges and management strategies for diabetes in children, the elderly, pregnant women, and individuals with other coexisting medical conditions.

Children with diabetes need tailored approaches to manage their blood sugar levels while supporting their growth and development. Elderly individuals often face complications due to other age-related health issues like high blood pressure, vision problems and arthritis making diabetes management more complex. Pregnant women with diabetes, whether pre-existing or gestational, require careful monitoring to ensure the health of both mother and baby. Those with other comorbidities, such as heart disease or kidney problems, need coordinated care to address multiple health concerns simultaneously.

CHILDREN AND ADOLESCENTS

Type 2 diabetes never occurs in babies, but obese children may develop it. Babies with type 1 diabetes can lose weight and show symptoms like vomiting and diarrhea, which can lead to a missed diagnosis. A sign of diabetes in babies is frequent urination, which can be noticed through frequent wet diapers. Unlike adults, children do not need strict blood sugar control, as avoiding low blood sugar (*hypoglycemia*) is crucial for them. The brain needs glucose, and a growing child's brain should not be deprived of it. The parents hence should take extreme care to avoid hypoglycemia in children.

Type 2 diabetes often appears around the age of 10 in obese children. In the late 1990s, only 3% of diabetes cases in adolescents in the United States belonged to T2DM, but now it is as high as 45%. T2DM is increasing in adolescents.

Children with low blood sugar might have nightmares or headaches at night, so a bedtime snack is important for them. Parents should ensure their children do not skip meals and encourage them to eat a snack before exercising.

Type 2 diabetes is more likely in an obese child than T1DM, and the symptoms might be less obvious. All overweight children should be screened for diabetes, especially those from high-risk ethnic groups. To prevent childhood obesity, women should exercise before and during pregnancy and avoid sugary drinks and fatty foods. Babies should be breastfed for at least six months. Children should be encouraged to stay active, and parents should set an example by exercising with them. Screen time, such as TV, video games, and computer games, should be limited.

<u>Growth and Development</u>

Diabetes can affect a child's growth and development in several ways. For example, managing diabetes during the critical periods of growth and puberty can be challenging because the body's needs keep changing significantly. Children with diabetes whose blood sugar is not well controlled might experience growth delays or other developmental problems. It is very important to monitor their growth and adjust their insulin doses and dietary plans to ensure they are growing normally and reaching the expected developmental milestones.

As children grow, their insulin requirements and dietary needs change. During puberty, insulin sensitivity can vary as the appetite increases. Parents and caregivers need to work with doctors to make necessary adjustments in insulin dosage and meal plans to support the child's healthy development and maintain stable blood glucose levels. This often involves regular consultations with a dietitian and frequent monitoring of blood glucose levels to make adjustments.

<u>Psychosocial Factors</u>

A diagnosis of diabetes can be overwhelming for children and adolescents. They might experience a range of emotions like fear, sorrow, or frustration. It is very important to provide emotional support and counseling at this stage to help them understand and cope with their condition. Support groups or counseling sessions can be beneficial for addressing the psychological impact of diabetes and helping children navigate their feelings.

Adolescents often face challenges with peer relationships and social acceptance, which can be complicated by their diabetes management. They might worry about how their condition affects their interactions with friends or their ability to participate in social activities. It is necessary to encourage open communication and provide guidance on how to manage diabetes in social situations, which helps them to build self-confidence and maintain healthy relationships with their peers. [See Chapter 7 on *Type 1 Diabetes mellitus*].

Managing diabetes while keeping up with schoolwork and extracurricular activities can be often demanding. Children need to balance their diabetes care, such as checking blood glucose levels and administering insulin, with their daily routines. Schools and extracurricular programs should be informed and supportive, providing accommodation where necessary. Parents and caregivers need to work with teachers and coaches to create a supportive environment that helps children manage their diabetes while participating in school and recreational activities.

<u>Education and Empowerment</u>

Diabetes education plays a crucial role in managing the condition effectively. Children and their families must understand the basics of diabetes, including how to manage blood glucose levels, administer insulin, and make healthy food choices. As the children grow up, they should be taught how to take care of themselves and understand their condition, making them active participants in their diabetes management.

As children grow, they should learn how to monitor their blood glucose levels, self-administer insulin injections or use insulin pumps, and count carbohydrates. Parents and caregivers should work on gradually increasing the child's responsibilities, encouraging them to take on more tasks as they become capable. This involves teaching them how to handle their diabetes management tasks, such as adjusting insulin doses, handling diabetes supplies, and recognizing symptoms of high or low blood sugar. This helps build confidence and prepares them for managing their diabetes as they move into adulthood.

This involves teaching them how to handle their diabetes management tasks, such as adjusting insulin doses, handling diabetes supplies, and recognizing symptoms of high or low blood sugar. This helps build confidence and prepares them for managing their diabetes as they move into adulthood.

Management Strategies

<u>Insulin Therapy</u>

Insulin needs of children change, especially during growth spurts and increased physical activity. During a growth spurt, a child's body needs more insulin to manage blood glucose levels effectively. Also, physical activities, such as sports or running, can affect how the body processes insulin. Hence, it becomes important to adjust insulin doses accordingly to accommodate these changes. This requires close monitoring and regular consultations with doctors to ensure that insulin doses are appropriate for the child's current growth and activity levels.

Insulin therapy for children and adolescents can be managed through different methods, including insulin pumps and multiple daily injections. Insulin pumps provide a continuous supply of insulin. On the other hand, multiple daily injections involve giving insulin using syringes or pens several times a day. Each method has its own advantages, and the choice depends on the child's lifestyle, preferences, and medical needs. Working with a healthcare team helps determine the most effective insulin delivery method for one's child.

Physical activities can cause blood glucose levels to drop, leading to hypoglycemia. To prevent this from occurring, it is important to monitor blood glucose levels closely before, during, and after sports or other physical activities. Children should be taught how to recognize the signs of hypoglycemia and how to manage it, such as by consuming a quick source of glucose if needed. They should be directed to carry glucose tablets or candies with them always. Having a plan in place for managing blood sugar during physical activities helps ensure that children stay safe and enjoy their activities without undue worry.

<u>Diet and Nutrition</u>

Dietary needs for children and adolescents with diabetes should be adjusted to their age and developmental stage. Younger children have different nutritional needs compared to teenagers, and it is important to provide them with balanced meals that support their growth and energy levels. Dietary recommendations should include a mix of carbohydrates, proteins, and fats, and take into account the child's personal preferences and cultural practices. Working with a dietitian helps to create a meal plan that meets these needs while managing blood glucose levels effectively. One of the key aspects of diabetes management is balancing carbohydrate intake with insulin doses. Carbohydrates impact blood glucose levels, so it is important to count carbohydrates and adjust insulin doses accordingly. This involves teaching children and their families how to estimate carbohydrate content in meals and snacks and how to adjust insulin doses based on this information. By understanding how different foods affect blood glucose levels, children learn to make sensible choices and maintain better control over their diabetes.

Special occasions, such as birthdays or holidays, can pose challenges for diabetes management due to the presence of treats and indulgent foods. It is important to plan ahead and make adjustments to insulin doses or meal plans to accommodate these occasions. Children should be encouraged to enjoy treats in moderation while maintaining good blood glucose control. Strategies include planning the dose of insulin or choosing healthier options, so that children can participate in celebrations without feeling deprived. Children should be encouraged to make sensible choices without feeling distressed or deprived.

<u>Continuous Glucose Monitoring (CGM)</u>

Continuous Glucose Monitoring (CGM) offers several benefits for children and adolescents with diabetes. CGMs provide real-time information about blood glucose levels throughout the day and night, which helps in maintaining better control. CGMs can help identify patterns and trends, making it easier to adjust insulin doses and meal plans as needed. This can lead to improved overall diabetes management and reduce the risk of both high and low blood sugar levels.

One of the significant advantages of CGMs is their ability to alert users to high or low blood glucose levels before they become severe. This proactive monitoring can help prevent episodes of hypoglycemia and hyperglycemia. Children may miss recognizing these symptoms. By providing alerts and trends, CGMs help in taking timely actions to correct glucose levels and avoid potential complications.

CGMs offer real-time data that can be accessed by parents and caregivers, thus allowing them to monitor their child's blood glucose levels at all times. This helps parents stay informed and involved in their child's diabetes management. Many CGMs have smartphone apps or remote monitoring capabilities, which helps caregivers to receive alerts and make adjustments as needed. This additional support helps ensure that children receive timely interventions and guidance to manage their diabetes effectively.

<u>Support Systems</u>

Family members and caregivers play a crucial role in supporting children with diabetes. They help in managing diabetes by helping with blood glucose monitoring, administering insulin, and providing emotional support. A supportive environment at home is essential for the child's well-being and diabetes management. Family members should work together to establish routines, provide encouragement, and offer practical assistance to help the child manage his condition effectively.

Schools too play an important role in the daily lives of children with diabetes. It is important to work with school personnel to ensure that the child's needs are met while at school. Teachers and school nurses should be informed about the child's diabetes management plan, arranging for necessary accommodations, and ensuring that staff are trained to handle diabetes-related situations, such as hypoglycemic episodes. Collaboration with school staff helps create a safe and supportive environment for the child during school hours.

Access to pediatric diabetes specialists, such as endocrinologists and diabetes educators, is important in the management of diabetes in children and adolescents. These specialists provide expert guidance and support in managing the condition and making treatment adjustments. In addition, joining support groups for families of children with diabetes can provide valuable emotional support, practical advice, and shared experiences. Support groups offer a sense of community and can help families navigate the challenges of managing diabetes.

ELDERLY INDIVIDUALS

As people grow older, their bodies undergo various changes which can affect the management of diabetes. For example, aging by itself often leads to reduced kidney function, which can impact how the body processes and eliminates medications and waste products, including those related to diabetes management. Also, metabolism generally slows down with age, hence, the body's ability to process glucose and insulin changes. Cognitive decline, or difficulties with memory and thinking, can also make it harder for older adults to manage their diabetes effectively by themselves. These age-related changes require adjustments in diabetes care so that blood sugar levels are managed appropriately, and complications are minimized.

Older adults with diabetes are at a higher risk for developing complications due to the natural aging process combined with the effects of diabetes. Cardiovascular disease (**CVD**) becomes more common as people age, and diabetes can aggravate this risk. CVD stands as the leading cause of death among individuals with diabetes. People with diabetes face a *2–4 times higher risk* of developing heart disease compared to those without the condition. The risk of heart disease increases significantly the longer a person lives with diabetes, making proactive management of both diabetes and cardiovascular health essential.

Diabetic Neuropathy, which causes nerve damage that can lead to pain or loss of sensation, is another concern in the elderly. Careful monitoring and preventive measures are needed to reduce the likelihood of serious health issues, such as heart attacks, strokes, or severe nerve damage.

Many elderly individuals have more than one health condition, such as high blood pressure (*Hypertension*) or arthritis, in addition to diabetes. Managing these multiple conditions requires an approach that addresses each of these issues without causing conflicts or complications. Medications used to treat hypertension or arthritis must be carefully chosen to avoid interactions with diabetic medications. Coordination between healthcare providers is crucial to ensure that all health problems are managed effectively and that treatments do not conflict with one another.

Furthermore, elderly individuals often take multiple medications for various health conditions; this is known as *Polypharmacy*. While these medications can be beneficial, they also come with risks, such as potential side effects or interactions between drugs. Managing diabetes alongside other medications requires careful monitoring and adjustments to avoid adverse effects. Doctors need to review all medications taken by the patient regularly to ensure that they are necessary, effective, and safe when used together.

<u>Functional Limitations</u>

Many older adults have difficulty in moving, which can affect their ability to engage in physical activities independently and perform daily self-care tasks. Hence, they may not be able to exercise regularly — an important requirement for managing diabetes. Difficulties with mobility can also affect the ability to manage diabetes care tasks, such as preparing healthy meals or accessing healthcare services, especially when they are living alone. Finding ways to adapt diabetes management practices to overcome these limitations is essential for maintaining health and well-being.

Aging often leads to vision problems, such as decreased visual acuity, and decreased dexterity, which affects the ability to handle small objects. This difficulty may be compounded by the presence of arthritis of the finger joints. This can make it difficult for older adults to monitor their blood glucose levels accurately or to administer insulin injections themselves. Hence using assistive devices, such as larger-print blood glucose meters or insulin pens with easier-to-use features may be necessary. Such user-friendly diabetic management tools can help older adults maintain control over their diabetes despite their physical limitations. They should seek the advice of their healthcare providers if they face such problems in management.

<u>Management Strategies</u>

For elderly individuals, managing diabetes can become overwhelming, especially when there are multiple medications and complex routines. Simplifying treatment plans can make it easier for older adults to follow their routines. Reducing the number of medications that they take, choosing medications that are easier to use, and simplifying dosing schedules are some ways to help them follow their routines without problem. *In many countries like India, combination medications are available. These provide a convenient dosing for the elderly by reducing the number of tablets to be taken.*

Older adults are more vulnerable to the dangers of hypoglycemia, which can cause dizziness, confusion, and even fainting. They become more prone to falls due to this. To minimize this risk, doctors often prescribe medications that are less likely to cause hypoglycemia. This makes diabetes management safer and reduces the chances of serious complications.

Furthermore, blood glucose targets are also tailored to each individual's overall health and lifestyle. For older adults, this might mean *aiming for slightly higher blood glucose levels to avoid the risk of hypoglycemia*. These targets should be set in consultation with the patient's doctor, taking into account the person's age, physical condition, and other health issues.

<u>Diet and Nutrition</u>

The dietary needs and preferences of the elderly often change. Ensuring that an elderly person's diet is both nutritious and enjoyable is crucial for their overall health and well-being. This involves including foods they like but at the same time meet their nutritional requirements without causing blood glucose spikes.

Proper nutrition is essential for managing diabetes, but it can be challenging to balance blood glucose control with getting enough nutrients. Elderly individuals need to consume a diet that provides all necessary vitamins and minerals while also keeping blood glucose levels stable. This often requires careful planning and the guidance of a dietitian.

Older adults are at a higher risk of malnutrition and unintended weight loss, which can complicate diabetes management. This is especially so in those living alone as they often have a tendency to skip meals making them more prone not only to malnutrition, but also to hypoglycemic episodes. Ensuring they consume enough calories and nutrients is important. Regular meals and snacks that are balanced and nutrient-dense can help prevent these issues. Whenever needed, nutritional supplements may be given to the elderly on the advice of the physician.

<u>Monitoring and Safety</u>

Regular monitoring of blood glucose levels is essential to detect hypoglycemia and other potential complications early. This involves routine blood tests using a glucometer or the use of CGMs that provide ongoing blood sugar readings. Continuous glucose monitors can be particularly helpful for elderly individuals because they provide real-time blood glucose data and alerts for high or low levels. It can be monitored by caregivers also. Simplified devices with larger displays and easier operation make self-monitoring more manageable for those with vision or dexterity issues.

Since hypoglycemia can cause dizziness and disorientation increasing the risk of falls and injuries in elderly individuals, safety measures, such as keeping living spaces free of hazards, using assistive devices for mobility, and ensuring timely treatment of low blood sugar episodes, are crucial for preventing accidents.

Since hypoglycemia can cause dizziness and disorientation increasing the risk of falls and injuries in elderly individuals, safety measures, such as keeping living spaces free of hazards, using assistive devices for mobility, and ensuring timely treatment of low blood sugar episodes, are crucial for preventing accidents.

<u>Support Systems</u>

Family members and caregivers play a vital role in supporting elderly individuals with diabetes. Their involvement can include helping with medication administration, meal planning, and monitoring blood glucose levels. This support can ensure better adherence to diabetes management routines.

Community resources and Senior Care Programs can provide additional support and services for elderly individuals with diabetes. These might include Meal delivery programs, Transportation services, and Social activities that promote overall well-being and independence. Many elderly individuals face social isolation and mental health challenges, which can negatively impact their diabetes management. Connecting them with social groups, counseling services, and mental health resources can help address these issues, providing emotional support and enhancing their quality of life.

In many Asian cultures like India and China, the joint family system or the extended family is still prevalent in numerous communities and societies. Within this traditional setup, the elderly are cared for by the entire family, which helps mitigate many issues that are more common in Western societies. The elderly are better cared for in these close knit societies. However, as the nuclear family system becomes more widespread in the East, new challenges for the elderly are emerging. This shift is particularly problematic in areas lacking advanced medical facilities. With fewer family members available to provide support and care, elderly individuals face increased risks and difficulties. Consequently, the move away from the joint family system is beginning to expose the elderly to problems previously uncommon in these cultures, highlighting the need for improved healthcare infrastructure and social support systems to address these evolving needs.

PREGNANT WOMEN

In the United States, 0.4% of pregnancies occur in women who already have diabetes, while 9.2% of women develop diabetes during pregnancy. Women with diabetes who are planning to become pregnant should aim to lose weight, quit smoking, manage high blood pressure, and switch to insulin under their doctor's guidance. All pregnant women are routinely checked for diabetes during their pregnancy.

The National Vital Statistics System (**NVSS**) has reported a notable rise in the percentage of mothers diagnosed with gestational diabetes mellitus (**GDM**) in the United States. The percentage increased from 6% in 2016 to 8.3% in 2021. Additionally, the incidence of GDM appears to correlate with maternal age. In 2021, mothers aged 40 and older had a GDM rate of 15.6%, whereas the rate for mothers under the age of 20 was significantly lower at 2.7%. This trend highlights the increasing risk of GDM with advancing maternal age and underscores the importance of monitoring and managing blood sugar levels during pregnancy, especially for older expectant mothers. The data emphasizes the need for awareness and preventive measures to manage this growing health concern among pregnant women.

Gestational Diabetes

Gestational diabetes (GDM) is diabetes that develops for the first time during pregnancy. This has already been discussed in detail in Chapter 6 on *Gestational Diabetes*. Several risk factors can increase a woman's likelihood of developing this condition, such as being overweight, having a family history of diabetes, or being older than 25 during pregnancy. Doctors screen for gestational diabetes using specific tests, usually between the 24th and 28th weeks of pregnancy, to ensure early detection and management.

Gestational diabetes can have significant effects on both the mother and the baby. For the mother, it can increase the risk of high blood pressure and *Preeclampsia* – a serious complication in pregnancy that is detrimental to both mother and baby. For the baby, GDM can lead to birth complications such as being significantly larger than average (*Macrosomia*), which can cause difficulties during delivery. Additionally, babies born to mothers with GDM are at higher risk of developing diabetes later in life.

<u>Pre-Existing Diabetes</u>

Women who already have Type 1 or Type 2 diabetes face unique challenges when they become pregnant. Managing blood glucose levels becomes even more crucial to ensure a healthy pregnancy. The woman needs more frequent blood glucose monitoring and adjustments in diabetes management routines.

Poor control of blood glucose levels during pregnancy can lead to serious complications. These include birth defects (*Congenital anomalies*), babies born too early (*Prematurity*), and preeclampsia. Ensuring good glucose control is absolutely mandatory to reduce these risks and promote a healthy pregnancy for both mother and baby. Miscarriages may occur if the diabetes is not properly controlled.

Management Strategies

<u>Blood Glucose Monitoring</u>

During pregnancy, it is very important to keep blood glucose levels within a specific range to protect both the mother and the baby. This requires frequent monitoring of blood glucose levels, often several times a day. Regular monitoring helps in making timely adjustments to diet, exercise, and medication.

Continuous Glucose Monitors (**CGMs**) can be very helpful during pregnancy. These devices provide real-time data on blood glucose levels and show trends over time, making it easier to manage glucose levels and make necessary adjustments promptly.

<u>Insulin Therapy</u>

Insulin needs can vary significantly during pregnancy due to hormonal changes occurring in the mother. This affects the way the body uses insulin. Hence, it is essential to adjust insulin doses regularly to keep blood glucose levels stable. The dose may have to be increased or decreased or the timing of insulin administration may have to be changed.

Both insulin pumps and multiple daily injections can be used safely during pregnancy. Insulin pumps deliver continuous insulin and can be adjusted easily, while multiple daily injections allow for flexibility in managing blood glucose levels. Both methods require careful monitoring and regular adjustments.

<u>Diet and Nutrition</u>

Pregnant women need to ensure they get enough nutrients for both themselves and their growing babies. This involves eating a balanced diet with the right amounts of carbohydrates, proteins, and fats. Adequate nutrition is crucial for the baby's development and the mother's health. Managing carbohydrate intake is essential for controlling blood glucose levels. Pregnant women need to balance the amount of carbohydrates they eat with their insulin doses and physical activity levels to maintain stable blood glucose levels. Healthy weight gain is a normal part of pregnancy, but excessive weight gain can cause complications. Pregnant women need to follow guidelines for healthy weight gain, which include eating nutritious foods and engaging in regular physical activity like walking.

<u>Medical Supervision</u>

Ongoing medical supervision is vital during pregnancy, especially for women with diabetes. Regular prenatal visits with a team of healthcare providers, including obstetricians, endocrinologists, and diabetes educators, help monitor the health of both mother and baby. Regular check-ups and ultrasound examinations help ensure that the baby is growing and developing as expected. Monitoring fetal growth allows healthcare providers to detect and address any problems early.

Planning for delivery involves discussing the safest delivery options and preparing for any potential complications. Postpartum care includes monitoring the mother's blood glucose levels after delivery and adjusting diabetes management as needed. It also involves ensuring the baby's health and monitoring for any signs of low blood glucose levels (*hypoglycemia*) in the newborn.

PEOPLE WITH COEXISTING MEDICAL CONDITIONS

Many people with diabetes also suffer from other health conditions such as high blood pressure, heart disease, kidney problems, and mental health issues. These additional conditions can complicate the management of diabetes. It is important to realize how diabetes medications interact with treatments for other health conditions. Some medications might affect how diabetes drugs work or cause side effects that need careful management.

<u>Complex Treatment Plans</u>

When a person has multiple health conditions, managing all treatments together can be complex and pose a challenge. It is essential to ensure that the management of diabetes does not interfere with the treatment of other conditions. Taking multiple medications (*Polypharmacy*) can increase the risk of side effects and interactions between drugs. This requires careful monitoring and coordination between healthcare providers.

<u>Management Strategies</u>

Effective management requires a team approach, where doctors, nurses, dietitians, and other healthcare professionals work together. This ensures that all aspects of the patient's health are addressed. Creating a treatment plan that considers all of the patient's health problems helps in managing diabetes along with other conditions. This includes regular check-ups and assessments. Continuous monitoring and adjustments to the treatment plan are necessary to accommodate changes in the patient's health status. This helps in maintaining balanced care for all conditions.

<u>Medication Management</u>

Regular reviews of all medications the patient is taking helps to identify and minimize harmful interactions. Adjustments should be made to ensure that the various medications work well together. Choosing medications that are effective for diabetes and also beneficial for other conditions can simplify treatment and reduce risks. For example, some medications given for diabetes can also help with weight loss or lower blood pressure. Keeping a close watch on side effects and potential complications from medications ensures timely intervention and management, reducing the risk of serious health issues. When multiple doctors are managing the patient for various illnesses, they should all be informed of all the medications that the patient is taking.

<u>Lifestyle Modifications</u>

Developing a diet and exercise plan that addresses the needs of diabetes and other health conditions helps in overall health management. This includes considering dietary restrictions and physical capabilities. Methods to overcome challenges to physical activity, such as mobility issues, ensure that the patient can stay active within their limitations. Encouraging a healthy lifestyle choice beyond diet and exercise, such as quitting smoking and managing stress, supports overall health and improves the management of multiple conditions.

<u>Patient Education and Support</u>

Educating patients about how to manage their diabetes along with other health conditions empowers them to take control of their health. This includes understanding the importance of each treatment and how they work together. Connecting patients with support groups and resources for diabetes and other health conditions provides emotional support and practical advice. This helps patients feel less isolated and more supported. Teaching patients how to monitor their health, manage their medications, and make healthy lifestyle choices encourages independence and self-confidence in managing their conditions.

Chapter 12 - MEDICATIONS IN DIABETES

Managing diabetes often requires medication to keep blood sugar levels in check. This chapter will guide the diabetic through the various types of medications used to treat diabetes, their purposes, and how to use them safely and effectively. It is crucial to understand that diabetes medications should only be started or changed under the guidance of a healthcare professional. Self-medication can lead to serious health complications.

When taking diabetes medications, one should follow the doctor's instructions precisely. This includes knowing the correct dosage, the best times to take the medicine, and whether it should be taken with food, before food or after food. Consistency in taking the medication is key to maintaining stable blood sugar levels.

Additionally, it is essential to be aware of any potential side effects and interactions with other drugs one may be taking. Regular check-ups with one's doctor will help monitor progress and make necessary adjustments to the treatment plan.

Patient education plays a vital role in diabetes management. Understanding one's medications, their role in treatment, and the importance of adherence can significantly improve the quality of life. Always one should communicate openly with the healthcare team about any concerns or questions they have regarding medications.

ORAL MEDICATIONS

An array of oral medications is used in the management of diabetes. They are discussed in brief below. By understanding the different types of oral diabetes medications and how they work, individuals with diabetes can better manage their condition and work with their healthcare providers to find the best treatment plan for their needs. It is important for the patients to understand the details of the medications that they are taking and be familiar with its side effects and dosage.

Biguanides (e.g. Metformin)

Biguanides, such as Metformin, primarily work by reducing the amount of glucose that the liver releases into the bloodstream. Additionally, they help the muscles use insulin more effectively, which helps to lower blood sugar levels. Metformin is often the first medication doctors prescribe for people with T2DM. It is known for being very effective in controlling blood sugar levels. One of the major benefits of Metformin is that it can help lower blood sugar without causing weight gain, rather it can also help with weight loss, which is an added advantage for many people with diabetes.

Sulfonylureas (e.g., Glipizide, Glyburide, Glimepiride)

Sulfonylureas help by stimulating the pancreas to produce more insulin. This extra insulin helps lower blood sugar levels. These medications are often used in combination with other diabetes medications to enhance blood sugar control. Sulfonylureas are effective at lowering blood sugar levels quickly, making them a good option for immediate blood sugar control.

Meglitinides (e.g., Repaglinide, Nateglinide)

Meglitinides stimulate the pancreas to release insulin, but they do so in a rapid and short-acting manner. This means they help control blood sugar levels immediately after eating. These medications are particularly useful for managing blood sugar spikes that occur right after meals.

Thiazolidinediones (TZDs) (e.g., Pioglitazone, Rosiglitazone)

Thiazolidinediones, or TZDs, work by making the body's cells more sensitive to insulin. They help fat, muscle, and liver cells use insulin more effectively, which lowers blood sugar levels. TZDs are effective in lowering blood sugar levels and have a long-lasting effect, which means they can help maintain stable blood sugar over time. These can cause weight gain.

DPP-4 Inhibitors (e.g., Sitagliptin, Saxagliptin, Linagliptin)

DPP-4 inhibitors work by blocking the action of an enzyme called DPP-4. This increases the levels of certain hormones that help regulate blood sugar. These medications do not typically cause weight gain and have a low risk of causing hypoglycemia.

SGLT2 Inhibitors (e.g., Canagliflozin, Dapagliflozin, Empagliflozin)

SGLT2 inhibitors work by preventing the kidneys from reabsorbing glucose back into the bloodstream. Instead, the excess glucose is excreted in the urine. These medications can help with weight loss and lower blood pressure. They also provide cardiovascular benefits, which can be particularly important.

Alpha-glucosidase Inhibitors (e.g., Acarbose, Miglitol)

Alpha-glucosidase inhibitors slow down the absorption of carbohydrates in the intestine. This helps to prevent blood sugar spikes after meals. By reducing post-meal blood sugar spikes, these medications can help maintain more stable blood sugar levels throughout the day.

GLP-1 Receptor Agonists (e.g., Exenatide, Liraglutide)

GLP-1 receptor agonists mimic the action of a natural hormone called GLP-1. This hormone helps stimulate the release of insulin, reduce the release of *glucagon* (a hormone that raises blood sugar), and slow down the emptying of the stomach. These medications can promote weight loss and reduce the risk of cardiovascular events, providing additional health benefits beyond blood sugar control.

Side Effects and Interactions

Different medications can have different side effects. Understanding the potential side effects and interactions of diabetes medications is key to managing your health effectively.

Common Side Effects

Gastrointestinal Problems with Metformin: People taking Metformin may often experience stomach-related problems. These may include feelings of nausea and episodes of diarrhea. While these side effects are typically mild, they can be bothersome, especially when first starting the medication.

Hypoglycemia Risk: Medications like Sulfonylureas and Meglitinides can sometimes cause blood sugar levels to drop too low. This can make one feel shaky, dizzy, or even faint. It is important to be aware of this risk and know how to manage low blood sugar episodes.

Weight Gain and Fluid Retention: Some people taking Thiazolidinediones may notice they gain weight or experience swelling in the legs due to fluid retention. These side effects can be concerning and may require adjustments in diet or medication.

Genital and Urinary Infections: Medications like SGLT2 inhibitors can increase the risk of infections in the genital area and urinary tract. These infections can be uncomfortable and may require medical treatment to resolve. These medications cause the kidneys to excrete more glucose in urine. This can make the genital area more susceptible to bacterial growth and infection.

Serious Side Effects

Lactic Acidosis : Although it is very rare, Metformin can sometimes cause a serious condition called *Lactic Acidosis*. This is a buildup of lactic acid in the body and can be very dangerous. Symptoms include muscle pain, difficulty breathing, and feeling extremely tired. If these symptoms occur, it is important to seek medical attention immediately.

Cardiovascular Risks: Certain sulfonylurea medications may carry a risk of heart-related problems. This includes an increased chance of heart attacks or other cardiovascular issues. It is crucial to discuss these risks with one's healthcare provider.

Increased Risk of Bone Fractures: Taking thiazolidinediones can sometimes lead to weaker bones, making them more susceptible to fractures. This risk can be particularly significant for older adults or those with existing bone health issues.

Drug Interactions

Diabetes medications can sometimes interact with other drugs the patient may be taking. This includes medications for high blood pressure (*Antihypertensives*) or high cholesterol (*Lipid-lowering drugs*). These interactions can affect how well the diabetes medication works or increase the risk of side effects.

It is essential to let the doctors and pharmacists know about all the medications and supplements one is taking. This includes over-the-counter drugs and herbal remedies also, as they can also interact with diabetes medications.

Monitoring and Adjustments

Keeping a close watch on blood sugar levels is important to see how well the medication is working. Regular testing helps to identify any patterns or issues that might need addressing. The doctor may need to adjust the medication dosage based on the blood sugar readings and any side effects one experiences. This ensures the most benefit from the treatment while minimizing side effects. Regular check-ups with the healthcare team are crucial. These visits allow the doctor to monitor the patient's progress, make any necessary adjustments to the treatment plan, and address any concerns one might have.

INSULIN THERAPY

Various types of Insulin are available for the diabetic patient. It is important to have a working knowledge of the types of insulin available. Understanding these different types of insulin and how they work can help one manage diabetes more effectively. By understanding these types and working with one's healthcare provider, one can find the best way to manage diabetes effectively.

Types of Insulin

Rapid-Acting Insulin (e.g., Lispro, Aspart, Glulisine)

This type of insulin starts working very quickly, usually within 10 to 30 minutes after injection. Its maximum effect is between 30 to 90 minutes when it is injected. Its effects last for about 3 to 5 hours. Rapid-acting insulin is typically taken just before eating to help control blood sugar levels that spike after meals.

Short-Acting Insulin (e.g., Regular Insulin)

Short-acting insulin begins to work within about 30 minutes of taking it. It reaches its peak effect 2 to 3 hours after administration. The effects of this insulin last for approximately 5 to 8 hours. It is usually taken 30 to 60 minutes before a meal to help manage the increase in blood sugar that comes from eating.

Intermediate-Acting Insulin (e.g., NPH Insulin)

This insulin starts working 1 to 2 hours after injection. It has its maximum effect between 4 to 12 hours after administration. The effects can last for 12 to 18 hours. Intermediate-acting insulin is used to provide background insulin coverage throughout the day or night and is often taken twice daily.

<u>Long-Acting Insulin</u> (e.g., Glargine, Detemir)

It begins to work within 1 to 2 hours after injection. Long-acting insulin has a very minimal peak, meaning it does not have a significant period where it works more strongly than other times. The effects last up to 24 hours. This type of insulin is taken once daily to provide a steady level of insulin to help manage blood sugar levels throughout the day and night.

<u>Ultra-Long-Acting Insulin</u> (e.g., Degludec)

It starts working within 30 to 90 minutes after taking it. Ultra-long-acting insulin has no significant peak, providing a very stable level of insulin. Its effects can last for more than 24 hours. This insulin provides very long-lasting blood sugar control and allows for flexible dosing schedules, often only needing to be taken once a day.

Methods of Administration

There are several methods of administering insulin, each with its own benefits and considerations. They are briefly discussed below.

<u>Syringes and Vials</u>

The traditional method of administering insulin involves using a syringe and vial. This method has been used for many years and is still common today, especially in hospitals. The insulin is drawn into the syringe by inserting the needle into the vial and pulling back on the plunger. The syringe is checked to make sure there are no air bubbles. Air bubbles are removed by gently tapping the syringe to bring them to the top, then pushing the plunger slightly to remove them. The insulin is then injected just under the skin (*subcutaneously*). This is usually done in areas like the abdomen, thigh, or upper arm.

Insulin Pens

Insulin pens are a more convenient and easier-to-use alternative to syringes and vials. They are pre-filled (disposable) or refillable devices that make insulin administration simpler and more portable. To use an insulin pen, the needle is attached to the pen. The dose is dialed by turning the dial on the pen to the number of units one needs. The insulin is then injected subcutaneously by pressing the button on the end of the pen. This method is quick and straightforward, making it easier to manage insulin doses throughout the day. It is especially useful for elderly individuals who may not be able to draw insulin from a vial.

Insulin Pumps

Insulin pumps are advanced devices that deliver a continuous supply of insulin under the skin, providing a more consistent way to manage blood sugar levels. An insulin pump consists of the pump itself, tubing, and an infusion set. The pump is usually worn on the body, and it delivers insulin through the tubing to the infusion set, which is placed under the skin. One of the main advantages of an insulin pump is that it can deliver precise amounts of insulin continuously, which helps keep blood sugar levels more stable. It also offers greater flexibility in lifestyle, as it can adjust insulin delivery based on the patient's activities and meals.

Inhaled Insulin (e.g., Afrezza)

Inhaled insulin is a newer method of administering rapid-acting insulin, which is taken through the lungs. Inhaled insulin is taken before meals to help control blood sugar spikes that occur after eating. It works quickly because it is absorbed through the lungs and enters the bloodstream rapidly. While inhaled insulin is convenient for some, it may not be suitable for individuals with lung conditions, such as asthma or chronic obstructive pulmonary disease (COPD). It is important to discuss this with the doctor whether this method suits the patient.

<u>Adjusting Doses</u>

Many factors affect the insulin needs in the patient. These are briefly discussed below.

Factors such as diet, physical activity, stress, illness, and other medications can alter insulin needs. For example, eating more carbohydrates than usual or being less active can increase the patient's insulin requirements. Stress and illness, like a cold or the flu, can also raise blood sugar levels, necessitating more insulin. Regular blood glucose monitoring is crucial to understanding how these factors affect the blood sugar. By consistently checking the blood levels, the patient can identify patterns and make necessary adjustments to the insulin doses to keep the blood sugar within the target range.

<u>Basal Insulin:</u>

This type of insulin is long-acting and helps maintain steady blood glucose levels throughout the day and night. Adjusting basal insulin is essential for keeping fasting blood glucose levels within the desired range. If the patient's morning blood glucose readings are consistently high or low, it might indicate a need to adjust the basal insulin dose.

<u>Bolus Insulin:</u>

This is rapid-acting or short-acting insulin taken before meals to manage the rise in blood glucose after eating. Adjusting bolus insulin is necessary to cover the carbohydrates one consumes during meals and to correct high blood glucose levels. If one notices spikes in the blood glucose after meals, he might need to increase the bolus insulin dose.

An *Insulin-to-Carbohydrate ratio* is used to determine the amount of insulin needed per gram of carbohydrate consumed. For instance, a ratio might be 1 unit of insulin for every 10 grams of carbohydrates. This ratio can vary from person to person. To find one's ideal ratio, the patient might need to experiment under the guidance of a doctor. The doctor can help one track the blood glucose levels after meals and adjust the ratio based on how the body responds to the insulin and the carbohydrates that are consumed.

Professional Guidance

Adjusting insulin doses safely requires the expertise of healthcare providers. They can guide one on how to adjust the doses based on the blood glucose patterns, diet, and lifestyle changes. Regular follow-ups with the healthcare team are essential to ensure that the insulin regimen is working effectively.

During these follow-ups, the healthcare provider can review the blood glucose logs, discuss any patterns or concerns, and make necessary adjustments to the insulin doses. This collaborative approach helps maintain optimal blood glucose control and reduces the risk of complications.

Chapter 13 - SURGERY AND THE DIABETIC PATIENT

Having surgery can be stressful for a patient with diabetes. Diabetes has to be managed well before, during, and after surgery. This ensures smooth recovery and lowers the chances of complications. In this chapter, we will explain what a diabetic patient needs to know about preparing for surgery, what to expect during the surgery, and how to take care of themselves afterward. When a patient with diabetes goes for surgery, the body has trouble managing blood sugar levels as surgery is a stressful situation for the body. Surgery makes this even harder, so it is crucial to be well-prepared. Knowing what steps to take can aid in proper recovery. Below are given the steps which provide clear, easy-to-understand information for diabetic patients.

The stress induced by surgery, anesthesia, and illness leads to heightened secretion of counterregulatory hormones, such as cortisol, glucagon, growth hormone, and catecholamines which can increase blood sugar and cause hyperglycemia. Hyperglycemia is found to elevate morbidity and mortality risks, including delayed wound healing, an increased rate of infection, intensive care unit (ICU) admissions, prolonged hospital stays, and higher postoperative mortality.

First, we will discuss what one needs to do before the surgery. This includes consulting with one's doctor, adjusting the medications, and managing the blood sugar levels. Preparing well can help the patient feel more confident and reduce the risk of problems during and after the surgery.

Next, we will enumerate what happens on the day of the surgery. From arriving at the hospital to what one should bring with him; this will cover all the important details. Understanding what to expect can help ease the patient's anxiety and make the process smoother.

After the surgery, it is important to continue managing diabetes carefully. Tips on how to monitor one's blood sugar levels, take care of the wound and follow the doctor's instructions. Proper care after surgery is crucial for a good recovery. This knowledge will help them take better care of themselves and reduce the risks associated with surgery. Remember, being well-prepared is the key to a successful surgery and a smooth recovery.

Preparing for Surgery

<u>Consult Your Doctor</u>

Schedule an appointment with your doctor before your surgery to talk about how to manage your diabetes during this time. During this meeting, discuss your usual blood sugar levels, the medications you are currently taking, and any special instructions you might need to follow.

Some medicines might need to be changed or stopped for a while before the surgery to make sure everything goes smoothly. If you are taking aspirin or some other blood thinner which is prescribed to patients after a cardiac procedure like angioplasty, ask your doctor if it has to be stopped before surgery. Make sure that you understand exactly what your doctor wants you to do. These medicines increase the risk of bleeding. Oral diabetic medications may be stopped by the doctor 24 to 48 hours before surgery and the patient switched over to insulin for better control of blood sugar during and after surgery.

<u>Coordinate with the Surgical Team</u>

Make sure the surgeons and nurses know you have diabetes and tell them about any complications you have had because of diabetes. Let them know what your normal blood sugar levels are and how you usually manage your diabetes. Be ready for your diabetes management plan to change because of the surgery. The surgical team might have specific instructions for you to follow.

<u>Blood Sugar Management</u>

Check your blood sugar levels often in the days before your surgery. Keeping your blood sugar within the target range is important because high or low levels can affect how well you recover from surgery.

Follow your doctor's advice on how to adjust your insulin doses before and after surgery. You might need to be extra careful with your insulin and blood sugar checks during this time.

<u>Diet and Hydration</u>

Stick to any special diet instructions your healthcare team gives you. You might need to fast or follow a specific diet before the surgery.

Make sure you drink enough fluids as advised by your healthcare team. Drinking enough water can help keep your blood sugar levels stable and help you recover better after surgery.

Day of the Surgery

<u>Arrival and Preparation</u>

Make sure to arrive at the hospital or surgical center early, as directed by your healthcare team. This gives you plenty of time to complete check-in procedures and get ready for your surgery without feeling rushed.

Pack a bag with all the diabetes supplies you might need. This includes your blood glucose monitor, insulin, and any snacks you might need in case your blood sugar gets too low. Having these items on hand can help you feel more prepared and less anxious.

Patients with diabetes are often scheduled for surgery early in the day as they will be fasting.

<u>Managing Blood Sugar During Surgery</u>

The medical team will keep a close eye on your blood sugar levels during the surgery. This monitoring is crucial to avoid complications.

Your insulin needs might change while you are in surgery. The medical team will manage your insulin based on your specific condition and the type of surgery you are undergoing. They will make sure you get the right amount to keep your blood sugar stable throughout the procedure.

Diabetes may increase the risk for certain problems during or after your surgery like:

- Infection after surgery, especially in the surgical wound.
- Slow healing of the wound.
- Fluid, electrolyte, and kidney problems.
- Heart problems may occur postoperatively in some patients.

After Surgery

<u>Post-Surgery Monitoring</u>

After surgery, it is very important to keep a close eye on your blood sugar levels. Surgery can cause changes in your blood sugar, so you should check it more often than usual to make sure it stays within a safe range.

Take all medications or insulin exactly as your doctor tells you. They will give you specific instructions on how to adjust your diabetes management after surgery, so be sure to follow their advice closely.

<u>Wound Care and Recovery</u>

Carefully follow the wound care instructions your surgeon gives you. Pay attention to your wound for any signs of infection, such as redness, swelling, or unusual discharge. Detecting any problems early can help prevent complications.

Stick to your doctor's advice about how much activity you should do while you recover. Ease back into your normal routine slowly and continue to manage your diabetes as part of your recovery.

<u>Diet and Hydration</u>

Follow any special dietary guidelines your healthcare team gives you for after surgery. Eating balanced meals can help keep your blood sugar stable and support your healing process.

Drink plenty of fluids to stay well-hydrated. Good hydration is important for recovery and for managing your blood sugar levels.

<u>Managing Diabetes-Related Complications</u>

Be on the lookout for any diabetes-related complications that could arise after surgery, such as slow healing wounds or changes in blood sugar levels. If you notice anything unusual, contact your healthcare provider right away.

If you have any questions or concerns about how to manage your diabetes after surgery, do not hesitate to reach out to your healthcare provider. They are there to help you navigate your recovery and ensure you stay healthy.

After surgery the patient in encouraged to move around in bed and get out of bed frequently if the surgeon permits. This is mainly to prevent bedsores which can occur by prolonged lying in one posture without changing position.

Tips for a Smooth Surgery Experience

- Proper planning and communication with your healthcare team are key to a successful surgery and recovery.
- Make sure to schedule an appointment with your doctor well before the surgery. Discuss your current diabetes management plan and ask any questions you have about how surgery might affect it.
- Talk to your doctor about any non-diabetic medications you are taking. Some might need to be adjusted or stopped temporarily before the surgery to avoid complications.

o Make a checklist of everything you will need on the day of the surgery, including your diabetes supplies and any necessary paperwork. This can help reduce stress and ensure you do not forget anything important.

o Understand the procedures and instructions related to your surgery and diabetes management.

o Take time to learn about the surgery you will be having. Ask your doctor or surgeon to explain the steps involved and what you can expect before, during, and after the procedure. Also ask about the type of anesthesia that will be used (local or general).

o Make sure you fully understand all instructions given to you by your healthcare team. This includes how to prepare for surgery, what to do the day of the surgery, and how to care for yourself afterward.

o Adhere to all pre-surgery and post-surgery instructions to minimize risks and promote a smooth recovery.

o Follow all guidelines about what to eat and drink before surgery. Your doctor might ask you to fast for a certain period, and it is important to stick to this schedule to avoid complications during surgery.

o After the surgery, follow all instructions about medication, wound care, and activity levels. This will help you heal faster and reduce the risk of infection or other complications.

o Keep a close watch on your blood sugar levels as instructed by your healthcare team. Surgery can cause fluctuations in blood sugar, so it is important to monitor it frequently and adjust your management plan as needed.

By following these guidelines, you can help ensure that your surgery goes as smoothly as possible and that your diabetes is well-managed throughout the process. Maintaining a positive outlook and staying informed about your health can significantly impact your recovery. Educate yourself about your condition and the surgical procedure to feel more confident and prepared. If you have any specific concerns or questions, always consult your healthcare provider for personalized advice and support. They can provide tailored guidance to help you navigate the surgery and recovery process effectively, ensuring the best possible outcome for your health and well-being.

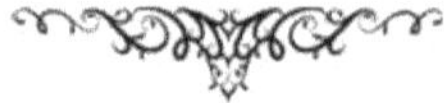

Chapter 14 - PSYCHOLOGICAL AND EMOTIONAL ASPECTS

Diabetes is not only a physical condition but also has significant psychological and emotional dimensions. Understanding these aspects is crucial for comprehensive diabetes management. Patients often face challenges such as stress, anxiety, and depression, which can affect their ability to manage their condition effectively. Emotional well-being plays a critical role in adherence to treatment plans, lifestyle modifications, and overall quality of life.

This chapter emphasizes the importance of patient education in addressing these psychological factors. By empowering patients with knowledge and coping strategies, we can foster a supportive environment that encourages better mental health and more effective diabetes management.

Impact of Diabetes on Mental Health

Stress and Anxiety

Managing diabetes involves a lot of daily tasks, such as checking blood sugar levels, counting carbohydrates, and taking medications. These tasks can become overwhelming and stressful, as they require constant attention and diligence. People with diabetes often worry about their blood sugar levels dropping too low or rising too high. Both conditions can be dangerous and cause immediate health problems. This can cause significant anxiety in them. Children and adolescents are more prone to worry about their condition as it often may interfere with their interaction with peers. Long-term complications such as heart disease, kidney problems, and nerve damage occur in diabetes. Knowledge about these and worrying about them can cause ongoing anxiety and stress in many patients. This is seen more in the middle aged and the elderly.

<u>Depression</u>

Patients with diabetes are more likely to experience depression compared to those without the condition. The daily demands of managing diabetes can contribute to feelings of sadness and hopelessness. Diabetes and depression often influence each other. Having diabetes can increase the risk of developing depression, and being depressed can make it harder to manage diabetes effectively. Depression in people with diabetes may manifest as a lack of motivation to manage their condition, changes in eating habits, and a general sense of despair about their health.

<u>Diabetes Distress</u>

A condition named *'Diabetes Distress'* has been described. It refers to the specific emotional burdens and worries that come with managing diabetes. This is different from general stress and anxiety because it is directly related to the challenges of living with diabetes. Many people with diabetes feel overwhelmed by the constant need to monitor their health. They may become frustrated with the unpredictability of their blood sugar levels and experience burnout from the never-ending demands of their condition. Diabetes distress is unique because it focuses solely on the emotional challenges associated with diabetes management, unlike general stress and anxiety which can stem from various aspects of life.

<u>Impact on Quality of Life</u>

Living with diabetes often requires making significant lifestyle changes, such as adhering to a strict diet, maintaining regular exercise, and avoiding certain activities that could affect blood sugar levels. These restrictions can limit one's freedom and spontaneity.

People with diabetes may feel different from their peers, especially when they need to check their blood sugar or administer insulin in social settings. This can lead to feelings of isolation and exclusion. Diabetes management can affect relationships with family and friends. Loved ones might worry about the person with diabetes or feel burdened by the additional care responsibilities. This can strain family dynamics and relationships.

<u>Eating Disorders</u>

People with diabetes, especially those who need to monitor their diet closely, may be at higher risk for developing disordered eating behaviors. Some patients may deliberately underuse insulin to lose weight. This is a serious concern. It is called *Diabulimia*. Strict dietary monitoring, often self-imposed, can lead to unhealthy attitudes towards food and issues regarding body image. Constant focus on what and how much to eat can contribute to an unhealthy relationship with food. Signs of eating disorders in people with diabetes may include frequent fluctuations in blood sugar levels, obsession with food and weight, avoiding insulin to lose weight, and severe anxiety around eating.

Coping Strategies and Support

<u>Education and Empowerment</u>

It is very important for patients with diabetes to learn about their condition and its effective management. This knowledge helps them understand what diabetes is, how it affects their body, and what they can do to stay healthy. Once patients are well-informed about their diabetes, they feel more confident and capable of managing it. This comes from knowing how to monitor blood sugar levels, make healthy food choices, and take medications correctly. Diabetes education programs are designed to teach people with diabetes everything they need to know about their condition. They provide practical tips and skills for managing diabetes on a daily basis, helping individuals take charge of their health. [See Chapter 16 on *Living with Diabetes*].

<u>Healthy Coping Mechanisms</u>

Managing stress is important for people with diabetes. Techniques like *Mindfulness, Meditation, Yoga* and *Relaxation exercises* can help reduce stress levels. These practices calm the mind and body, making it easier to handle the daily demands of diabetes. Regular physical activity is beneficial for both physical and mental health. Exercise helps to control blood sugar levels, improves mood, and reduces stress. Activities like walking, swimming, or yoga can be enjoyable ways to stay active. A balanced lifestyle includes getting enough sleep, eating a nutritious diet, and exercising regularly. [See Chapter 17 on *Exercise and Physical Activity Plans*]. These habits support overall well-being and make managing diabetes easier. Proper rest, healthy meals, and consistent physical activity create a strong foundation for health.

<u>Support Networks</u>

Having a supportive social network is vital for people with diabetes. Family and friends should offer emotional support, help with daily tasks, and provide encouragement to the patients, especially children and adolescents with diabetes. Special care should be taken not to let them feel ostracized. Their understanding and assistance make a big difference in managing diabetes. Where facilities are available, joining a support group with others who have diabetes can be very helpful. Sharing experiences and strategies with people who face similar challenges creates a sense of community and understanding. These groups can provide valuable tips and emotional support. Online communities, such as social media groups and forums, provide access to support and information. People with diabetes can connect with others, ask questions, and share their experiences. These virtual networks offer a convenient way to find support anytime. A diabetic patient should not be allowed to feel socially isolated.

<u>Professional Support</u>

Regular check-ups and open communication with healthcare providers are essential. Doctors, nurses, and diabetes educators can offer medical advice, adjust treatment plans, and answer any questions about managing diabetes. Open communication with them must be encouraged. Professional counseling or therapy can be very beneficial whenever needed. Cognitive-behavioral therapy (**CBT**) and other therapeutic approaches help people manage the emotional aspects of living with diabetes. Therapy provides tools to cope with stress, anxiety, and depression. Some support groups are led by healthcare professionals. These groups combine peer support with expert guidance, offering a well-rounded approach to diabetes management. Participants can share experiences and get professional advice.

<u>Practical Strategies</u>

Establishing a regular daily schedule for meals, medication, and blood sugar monitoring helps create consistency and predictability. A routine makes it easier to manage diabetes and ensures that important tasks are not forgotten. Setting achievable targets for blood glucose control and lifestyle changes is important. Realistic goals provide motivation and a sense of accomplishment. They help people make steady progress in managing their diabetes. Developing strategies to handle diabetes-related challenges and setbacks is crucial. Being prepared with solutions for common issues, like dealing with high or low blood sugar levels, helps individuals manage their condition more effectively and with less stress.

Role of Mental Health Professionals

<u>Identifying Mental Health Issues</u>

Mental health professionals play a crucial role in checking for signs of depression, anxiety, and emotional stress specifically related to diabetes during regular diabetes check-ups. They use special questionnaires and tools that can accurately identify mental health issues in patients with diabetes. These tools help in assessing the mental state of individuals with diabetes. It is very important to recognize these mental health issues early. Early detection and intervention can prevent these problems from becoming more serious and help to improve the overall well-being of the person.

<u>Integrated Care Approach</u>

This approach needs teamwork between the diabetes care team (like doctors and nurses) and mental health professionals (like psychologists and counselors). They work in unison to provide the best care for both the physical and mental health needs of the individual with diabetes. Combining expertise from different health professionals ensures that all aspects of a person's health are taken care of, leading to better overall health outcomes. Many integrated care programs have shown success in managing both diabetes and mental health, helping people live healthier and happier lives. These are available in many countries.

Therapeutic Interventions

This psychological therapy helps the patients change their negative thoughts and behaviors and teaches them how to think positively and act in healthier ways. Techniques like mindfulness and meditation help reduce stress and improve emotional control. Such therapy encourages individuals to accept their diabetes and commit to making positive changes in their lives.

Medication Management

Mental health professionals may occasionally prescribe medications to help manage mental health issues in patients with diabetes. These medications can be very helpful for individuals with diabetes who are also dealing with depression or anxiety. Interactions between diabetes medications and mental health medications should be carefully checked. Professionals ensure that these medications work well together without causing harm. Regular follow-ups are important to monitor how well the medications are working and to make any necessary changes to the treatment plan.

Family and Caregiver Support

The family members are also involved in therapy to help them understand the impact of diabetes and to improve family support. They offer information and resources to help caregivers support the individual with diabetes effectively. Professionals work on improving the relationships within the family to create a supportive and understanding environment for the person with diabetes.

<u>Community and Social Resources</u>

Mental health professionals help the patient to connect with community resources like support groups, educational programs, and social services that provide additional help and information. These organizations offer support, resources, and advocacy for people with diabetes. Engaging in community activities and volunteer opportunities can provide a sense of purpose and community, which is beneficial for mental health.

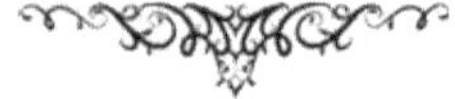

Chapter 15 - ADVANCED THERAPIES AND TECHNOLOGIES

*In recent years, significant advancements in diabetes care have led to the development of innovative therapies and cutting-edge technology. This chapter explores these advancements, which include Continuous Glucose Monitors (**CGMs**) that provide real-time blood sugar readings, Insulin Pumps that deliver precise doses of insulin, and Artificial Pancreas systems that automate blood sugar management. Emerging treatments and research in the field of diabetes are also highlighted, offering hope for even more effective diabetes control in the future.*

Patient education is crucial for utilizing these advanced technologies effectively. Understanding how to use these devices, their benefits, and potential challenges can empower the patients to manage their diabetes more efficiently. Staying informed and working closely with the healthcare team to incorporate these innovations into the diabetes care plan is advantageous to the patients and the caregivers.

Many of the advanced diabetes devices and technologies described below may not be available in many parts of the world. Even where they are available, the high cost can make them inaccessible to most patients. However, staying informed about these advancements is valuable for everyone with diabetes. Knowing about new developments can help individuals and their caregivers understand what might be possible in the future, even if they cannot access these resources right away.

Continuous Glucose Monitors (CGMs)

Continuous Glucose Monitors, commonly known as CGMs, are devices that keep track of one's blood glucose levels all day and night without needing frequent fingerstick tests. They provide a constant stream of data about the patient's blood sugar levels. These devices have a few essential parts: a small sensor that is introduced just under the skin, a transmitter that sends data from the sensor, and a receiver or display device like a smartphone or a specialized monitor that shows the glucose readings.

The sensor is designed to measure glucose levels in the fluid between the cells (*Interstitial fluid*). This is slightly different from the glucose in blood but gives a good estimate of blood sugar levels. The transmitter takes the information from the sensor and sends it to a receiver, which could be a separate device, a smartphone app, or even an insulin pump. This means the patient can see his glucose levels and trends in real-time. One of the best features of CGMs is their ability to provide continuous and real-time monitoring. The patients can see how the glucose levels change throughout the day and night, which helps them make better decisions about their diabetes management.

With real-time data, one gets immediate feedback on the blood glucose levels, helping him understand how his diet, exercise, and medications affect the glucose levels. CGMs can alert the patient with notifications if the glucose levels are too high or too low. This is especially helpful for preventing dangerous situations like hypoglycemia or hyperglycemia.

By providing detailed trends and patterns in the glucose levels, CGMs can thus help one maintain better overall glucose control, reducing the risk of complications and making day-to-day management of diabetes easier.

Some CGMs require periodic calibration with traditional fingerstick tests to ensure accuracy. This means the patient might still need to do some fingerstick tests to verify the CGM readings. CGMs are more expensive than traditional blood glucose monitors due to the higher upfront costs of the device and the ongoing cost of replacing sensors. Sensors for CGMs need to be replaced regularly, typically every 7 to 14 days, which adds to the ongoing maintenance and cost.

The *Dexcom G6* is a popular CGM that does not require calibration and can integrate with various insulin pumps and smartphone apps, making it a convenient option for many users. The *FreeStyle Libre* is known as a flash glucose monitoring system. Instead of continuous data streaming, one scans the sensor at intervals with a reader or smartphone to get the glucose readings.

The *Medtronic Guardian* works well with Medtronic's insulin pumps and can also be used as a standalone CGM, providing flexibility depending on your diabetes management needs.

Future CGMs are expected to offer improved accuracy and longer sensor wear times, reducing the need for frequent sensor replacements and calibrations. Research is ongoing to develop non-invasive glucose monitoring systems that do not require sensors to be placed under the skin, which would make glucose monitoring even more convenient and comfortable.

Insulin Pumps

Insulin pumps are small electronic devices that help people with diabetes manage their blood sugar levels by delivering insulin continuously throughout the day and night. Instead of taking insulin through multiple daily injections, insulin pumps provide a steady stream of insulin into the body. These devices consist of three main parts: the pump itself, which controls the delivery of insulin; the tubing, which connects the pump to the body; and the infusion set, which includes a tiny needle or cannula inserted under the skin to deliver insulin directly into the bloodstream.

Insulin pumps are designed to mimic the way a healthy pancreas works by delivering insulin in two ways. First, they provide a continuous, small amount of insulin called the *basal rate*. This helps maintain one's blood sugar levels at a steady baseline throughout the day and night. Second, they allow the patient to take larger doses of insulin, called *bolus doses*, at mealtimes. These doses help manage the rise in blood sugar that occurs when the patient eats carbohydrates. One of the great features of insulin pumps is that they can be customized to fit individual needs. The settings can be adjusted to deliver different amounts of insulin at different times of the day, based on the activity levels, meals, and blood sugar patterns of the patient.

Insulin pumps offer better control over blood sugar levels because they deliver insulin more precisely than injections. This can help the patient avoid both high and low blood sugar levels more effectively. They provide greater flexibility in daily life. One can easily adjust the insulin delivery for meals, exercise, and other activities, making it easier to maintain good blood sugar control. Many modern insulin pumps have advanced features, such as predictive algorithms and continuous glucose monitoring integration, which can help reduce the risk of hypoglycemia by predicting and preventing drops in blood sugar before they occur.

One of the main drawbacks of insulin pumps is the cost. They can be more expensive initially and over time, compared to traditional insulin injections. This includes the cost of the pump, supplies like tubing and infusion sets, and the need for regular replacements. Technical issues can also arise with insulin pumps. There is a potential for the pump to malfunction, or problems can occur at the infusion site, such as blockages or infections. Using an insulin pump effectively requires patient education and training. There is a learning curve to understanding how to set up the pump, adjust the settings, and troubleshoot any issues that might arise.

The *Medtronic MiniMed* is a popular insulin pump that can integrate with CGMs to provide a hybrid closed-loop system. This means it can automatically adjust insulin delivery based on the glucose levels.

The *Tandem t:slim X2* is another well-liked pump, known for its compact design. It can integrate with Dexcom CGMs, allowing for better glucose management through real-time data.

The *Omnipod* is a unique insulin pump system that is tubeless, making it more discreet and convenient to wear. It delivers insulin through a small pod that can be placed on different parts of the body.

Future insulin pumps are expected to offer more advanced closed-loop systems, which means they will automatically adjust insulin delivery based on continuous glucose monitor data. This can help maintain better blood sugar control with less manual intervention. Integration with smart devices is another exciting development. This will allow for remote monitoring and control of insulin pumps through smartphones or other smart devices, providing even greater convenience and ease of use.

Artificial Pancreas Systems

An artificial pancreas is a highly advanced medical device that aims to replicate the natural function of a healthy pancreas in regulating blood sugar levels. This system is also known as a closed-loop system because it continuously monitors and adjusts blood glucose levels without much input from the user. The system is made up of three main components: a continuous glucose monitor (CGM) that tracks glucose levels in real-time, an insulin pump that delivers insulin as needed, and a sophisticated control algorithm that calculates and administers the precise amount of insulin required to maintain optimal blood glucose levels.

The process begins with the CGM, which constantly measures the glucose levels in the fluid just beneath the skin. This data is sent to the control algorithm, a type of software that analyzes the information and predicts future glucose trends.

Based on the predictions, the control algorithm sends instructions to the insulin pump to either increase, decrease, or maintain the insulin delivery. This ensures that blood sugar levels stay within a healthy range throughout the day and night. The beauty of the artificial pancreas system lies in its automation. The user does not need to manually adjust insulin doses because the system continuously makes small adjustments in real-time, much like a healthy pancreas would.

One of the biggest advantages of using an artificial pancreas is the significant improvement in blood glucose control. These systems help keep glucose levels within the target range more consistently, reducing the risk of both high and low blood sugar episodes. Another major benefit is the reduction in hypoglycemia. The system can predict and adjust insulin delivery to prevent these dangerous lows. Additionally, artificial pancreas systems offer great convenience because users can spend less time managing their diabetes and enjoy a better quality of life.

Despite their benefits, artificial pancreas systems come with some limitations. One of the primary concerns is the cost. These devices are expensive, both in terms of the initial purchase and the ongoing maintenance. There are also technical challenges. The system relies on multiple components working together seamlessly, so there is always a risk of errors or malfunctions. Furthermore, these systems are still relatively new and not yet widely available. Access to artificial pancreas technology can be limited depending on geographic location, insurance coverage, and availability of the necessary components.

The *Medtronic MiniMed 670G* is one of the first hybrid closed-loop systems available. It automatically adjusts basal insulin delivery based on real-time glucose readings, although users still need to input carbohydrate counts for meals.

Another notable system is the *Tandem Control-IQ*, which pairs with the *Dexcom G6 CGM*. This system offers advanced algorithms for better glucose control and can adjust for both basal insulin and correction boluses.

In addition to commercial products, there are also DIY (do-it-yourself) systems like *Loop and OpenAPS*. These open-source projects are developed by the diabetes community and are used by tech-savvy patients who are comfortable building and maintaining their own systems.

Emerging Treatments and Research

<u>Beta Cell Replacement Therapy</u>

Scientists are working on developing new treatments that focus on replacing the insulin-producing cells in the pancreas - beta cells. One promising area of research involves using *Stem Cells* to create these beta cells in the lab. Stem cells are unspecialized cells which can transform themselves to any type of cells in the body. They are found in most parts of the body, including brain, bone marrow, blood vessels, skin, teeth and heart. By transforming stem cells into functioning beta cells, researchers hope to provide a new source of insulin for people with diabetes.

Another approach is called *Islet Transplantation*. This procedure involves taking clusters of pancreatic cells, called islets, from organ donors and transplanting them into people with diabetes thereby aiming to restore the body's ability to produce insulin naturally. While this technique shows promise, it currently faces challenges such as finding suitable donors and preventing the immune system from rejecting the transplanted cells.

<u>Gene Therapy</u>

Gene therapy is an exciting area of research that involves altering or repairing the genes responsible for diabetes. By targeting the root cause of the disease at the genetic level, scientists aim to develop long-term or even permanent treatments. These genetic modifications could potentially correct defects that lead to diabetes, allowing the body to regulate blood sugar levels more effectively. This innovative approach holds great promise for both Type 1 and Type 2 diabetes, offering hope for a future where the disease can be managed more effectively or even cured.

<u>Immunotherapy</u>

In Type 1 diabetes, the body's immune system mistakenly attacks and destroys insulin-producing beta cells. Immunotherapy aims to prevent or reverse this autoimmune attack. One approach involves using regulatory T cells or *Tregs* (white blood cells that regulate the immune system) to modulate the immune response and protect beta cells.

Another promising treatment is the use of *Anti-CD3 Monoclonal Antibodies*, which target specific parts of the immune system to prevent it from attacking beta cells. These therapies are still in the experimental stages, but they offer hope for preserving beta cell function and potentially halting the progression of Type 1 diabetes.

<u>Smart Insulin</u>

Imagine insulin that knows when to turn itself on or off based on your blood sugar levels. This is the idea behind smart insulin, also known as *Glucose-Responsive Insulin*. These innovative formulations are designed to activate when blood glucose levels are high and deactivate when levels are normal or low. The development of smart insulin could significantly reduce the risk of hypoglycemia. This would provide a more natural and safer way to manage diabetes, reducing the need for constant blood sugar monitoring and insulin adjustments.

<u>New Drug Classes</u>

Researchers are also exploring new classes of medications to improve diabetes management. One example is dual agonists, which target multiple pathways in the body to better control blood glucose levels. These drugs, such as GLP-1/GIP dual agonists, offer a more comprehensive approach to diabetes treatment.

Another exciting development is the potential use of SGLT2 inhibitors for managing Type 1 diabetes. Originally developed for Type 2 diabetes, these medications help the kidneys remove excess glucose from the body. Expanding their use to Type 1 diabetes could provide additional options for glucose control.

<u>Technological Innovations</u>

Advances in technology are opening new possibilities for diabetes management. Non-invasive glucose monitoring devices, which measure blood sugar levels without the need for needles or sensors, are being developed. These devices could make glucose monitoring less painful and more convenient.

Additionally, advanced wearables, such as *Smartwatches*, are being designed to track glucose levels along with other health metrics. These wearables could provide continuous, real-time data, helping individuals make more informed decisions about their diabetes management.

<u>Personalized Medicine</u>

Personalized medicine aims to tailor treatments based on an individual's unique genetic, environmental, and lifestyle factors. By understanding the specific characteristics of a person's diabetes, healthcare providers can customize therapies to achieve better outcomes.

Predictive analytics, which uses data to forecast the progression of diabetes and how individuals will respond to different treatments, is also an emerging field. This approach could lead to more effective and targeted treatment plans, improving the overall management of diabetes.

Chapter 16 - LIVING WITH DIABETES

Living with diabetes requires ongoing management and self-care to maintain a healthy and fulfilling life. This chapter will guide you through daily routines, from monitoring blood sugar levels to making informed food choices and staying active. We will explore practical tips for navigating the healthcare system, ensuring you receive the best possible care and support. Building a strong support network, including family, friends, and healthcare professionals, is essential for emotional and physical well-being. Many of the points highlighted in this chapter have already been discussed in various chapters of the book. The reader is requested to refer to the appropriate segments in various chapters while reading this short description on how to live with diabetes. This summary is a repetition of the things to be adopted by an individual who is diagnosed with the disease.

Additionally, this chapter will feature personal stories and testimonials from individuals living with diabetes, providing inspiration and real-life examples of how to thrive with this condition. Understanding and managing diabetes empowers you to lead a balanced, healthy life.

Daily Routines and Self-Care

<u>Morning Routine</u>

- Begin each morning by checking your blood sugar levels. This is important because it helps you understand how your body is doing and what steps you need to take for the day ahead.
- Choose a balanced breakfast that includes a mix of nutrients. Pay attention to the amount of carbohydrates, as these can affect your blood sugar levels. Proper carbohydrate counting can help keep your blood sugar steady.
- Make sure to take your morning medications and insulin if needed. It is crucial to follow the prescribed doses and take them at the right time to keep your diabetes under control.

<u>Meal Planning and Nutrition</u>

- Eat a variety of foods to get all the necessary nutrients. Control your portion sizes to avoid overeating. A balanced diet helps in maintaining steady blood sugar levels and overall health.
- Learn how to count carbohydrates and plan your meals accordingly. Eating at regular times can help manage your blood sugar levels more effectively.
- Choose snacks that will not cause your blood sugar to spike or drop suddenly. Some good options include nuts, fruits, and vegetables. [See Chapter 18 for *Nutritional Plans and Recipes*].

<u>Physical Activity</u>

- Regular physical activity is very important. It helps keep your blood sugar levels in check and improves your overall health.
- Include different kinds of exercises in your routine. Aerobic exercises like walking or cycling, resistance training like lifting weights, and flexibility and balancing exercises like stretching are all beneficial.
- Find practical ways to include physical activity in your daily life. This could be as simple as taking the stairs instead of the elevator, going for a walk after dinner or walking to the corner store to pick up groceries. [See Chapter 17 on *Exercise and Physical Activity Plans*].

<u>Monitoring Blood Glucose</u>

- Check your blood sugar levels multiple times a day if advised by your doctor. Do this before and after meals, and at bedtime, to keep track of how your body is responding. Maintain a record of the readings.
- Use blood glucose monitors or continuous glucose monitors (CGMs) to get accurate readings. Learn how to interpret the data to make informed decisions about your health.
- Maintain a diary of your blood sugar levels, what you eat, and your physical activities. This helps in understanding patterns and making necessary adjustments. Show it to your doctor when you go for the checkup. [See Chapter 9 on *Blood Glucose Monitoring*}.

<u>Medication and Insulin Management</u>

- There are different types of medications for diabetes, including pills, insulin, and other injectables. Having a basic knowledge of how each one works helps in managing your condition better.

- Store insulin properly to ensure it remains effective. Follow the guidelines for storage and handling to avoid any issues.

- Adjust your medication or insulin doses based on your blood sugar readings, what you eat, and your level of physical activity. This helps in maintaining better control over your diabetes. [See Chapter 12 on *Medications in Diabetes*].

Foot Care

- Inspect your feet every day for any cuts, blisters, or signs of infection. Early detection can prevent serious problems.

- Wear shoes that are comfortable and provide good support. Proper footwear can prevent injuries and complications. Always wear some form of footwear indoors. Never walk barefoot. Wear comfortable, preferably cotton socks with footwear.

- If you notice any problems with your feet, consult a healthcare provider right away. Prompt medical attention can prevent complications. [See Chapter 8 on *Complications of Diabetes- Foot care*].

Stress Management and Mental Health

- Practice techniques like mindfulness, meditation, and relaxation exercises to manage stress. Reducing stress can positively impact your blood sugar levels.

- Be aware of the signs of depression and anxiety. Managing your mental health is just as important as managing your physical health.

- Do not hesitate to seek help from counselors or join support groups. Talking to others who understand your challenges can provide comfort and practical advice.

[See Chapter 14 on *Psychological and Emotional Aspects*].

> *Edward, a 30-year-old salesman led a hectic lifestyle, starting his day at 7 a.m., traveling to meet clients, and often grabbing quick, unhealthy meals from roadside eateries. His breakfast was rushed, lunch typically consisted of a burger or sandwich paired with a soft drink, and his eating schedule was highly irregular. Lack of time for exercise and poor dietary choices led to a weight gain of ten pounds. During a routine check-up, he was diagnosed with type 2 diabetes, prompting a significant overhaul of his daily routine.*
>
> *Edward had to adopt a more structured approach to his meals, focusing on balanced, home-cooked options instead of fast food. He incorporated regular exercise into his daily schedule, such as brisk walking or jogging, and paid attention to portion sizes and timing of meals to maintain stable blood glucose levels. He also cut down on late-night work and social activities that interfered with his new, healthier lifestyle. These changes were essential to managing his diabetes and improving his overall well-being.*
>
> *Soon after making changes to his lifestyle, Edward noticed a significant transformation in his health. Within two months, he shed eight pounds, and his blood sugar levels were well-managed with oral medications. Along with this physical improvement, he also experienced a boost in energy, allowing him to thrive in his salesman's job. Having embraced these changes, he successfully adapted to life with diabetes, feeling more in control and optimistic about his future.*

Navigating Healthcare Systems

<u>Understanding Healthcare Coverage</u>

- There are different kinds of health insurance that people can have. Some get private insurance through their jobs or buy it themselves. Others might have Medicare if they are older, or Medicaid if they have lower income.
- It is important to know what your insurance covers when it comes to diabetes. This includes medications, supplies like test strips and insulin, and visits to specialists.
- Sometimes dealing with insurance can be tricky. Learn how to manage all the paperwork involved and know what to do if your insurance denies a claim. Understanding the appeal process can help you get the coverage you need.
- In countries like India, the insurance covers only patients admitted to hospital. Outpatient treatment is not covered by insurance. For those working in the government, reimbursement facilities are available for medications purchased on an outpatient basis.

<u>Choosing Healthcare Providers</u>

- Your main doctor, or primary care physician, plays a key role in helping you manage your diabetes. They keep track of your overall health and coordinate your care with other specialists.
- There are several specialists who can help with diabetes care. Endocrinologists specialize in diabetes and hormone-related issues. Dietitians can help you with meal planning. Podiatrists look after your feet, and Ophthalmologists take care of your eyes.

- It is important to have a team of healthcare professionals. Each one brings a different expertise to help you manage your diabetes in the best possible way.

Regular Check-Ups and Screenings

- Regular visits to your doctor and specialists are important. These appointments help monitor your condition and catch any problems early. Routine check-ups and specialist visits should be scheduled regularly.
- People with diabetes need certain screenings to stay healthy. These include HbA1c tests to monitor blood sugar control, eye exams to check for vision problems, foot exams to prevent complications, and kidney function tests. [See Chapter 9 on *Blood Glucose Monitoring*].
- Getting vaccinated is crucial. Flu shots and other vaccines are important because people with diabetes can be more vulnerable to infections.

Communicating with Healthcare Providers

Before your doctor's visit, keep a log of your symptoms, blood sugar readings, and any questions you might have. This helps you and your doctor have a more productive conversation.

Effective Communication:

- It is important to be open with your healthcare providers. Share your concerns and ask questions to understand your health better.
- Make sure you understand what your doctor is advising. Clarify any instructions about your treatment plan and know what you need to do for follow-up.

Accessing Diabetes Education and Resources

<u>Diabetes Self-Management Education (DSME) Programs</u>: These programs teach you how to manage your diabetes. They can be very beneficial, and knowing how to enroll can give you access to a lot of useful information.

<u>Online Resources and Tools:</u> There are many reliable websites, mobile apps, and online forums where you can find information and support about diabetes. These can be great tools to help you manage your condition.

<u>Community Resources:</u> Look for local support groups and diabetes education centers. These resources can provide support, information, and a sense of community with others who understand what you're going through. [See Chapter 20 on *Resources and Support*].

Building a Support Network

<u>Family and Friends</u>

- It is important to help your family and friends understand what diabetes is and how it is managed. The more they know about it, the better they can support you.
- Get your family involved in your care by planning meals together, exercising as a group, and providing emotional support. This can make managing diabetes easier and less lonely. Going for a morning walk with one's spouse is a good way of consolidating relationships while helping your blood sugar values.
- Be open about your needs. Let your family and friends know how they can help you. Whether it is reminding you to take your medication, helping with diet choices, or simply being there to listen, clear communication is key.

Peer Support Groups

- Joining a support group allows you to share your experiences with others who understand what you are going through. You can exchange tips and offer each other encouragement.
- Look for support groups in your local community centers, hospitals, or online. Many groups meet regularly to discuss various aspects of living with diabetes.

- Get involved in the activities offered by these groups, such as meetings, workshops, and social events. This can help you learn more and feel more connected. [See Chapter 20 on *Resources and Support*].

<u>Online Communities</u>

The internet has many forums and social media groups where you can connect with people who have diabetes. These platforms provide a lot of support and information. Participate actively by asking questions and sharing your own experiences. This can help you get new ideas and feel supported. Make sure to protect your privacy when you are online. Be cautious about sharing personal information and be wary of misinformation.

Professional Support

<u>Role of Diabetes Educators</u>: Diabetes educators are professionals who can provide you with detailed education about managing your condition. They offer personalized advice that can help you stay healthy.

<u>Counselors and Therapists</u>: Sometimes, managing diabetes can be stressful. Counselors and therapists can help you deal with the emotional and psychological aspects of the disease.

<u>Financial Advisors</u>: Diabetes care can be expensive. Financial advisors can help you manage the costs and find resources to make your care more affordable.

Personal Stories and Testimonials

<u>Inspiring Stories</u>

Learn about the journeys of people who have diabetes. Read about their challenges, how they faced them, and the triumphs they achieved along the way. Discover how people manage their diabetes every day, overcoming various hurdles to lead happy and fulfilling lives. These stories show that with determination, diabetes can be managed well.

Celebrate the successes of individuals with diabetes. From health improvements to career advancements and personal achievements, these stories highlight the many milestones reached despite the condition.

<u>Lessons Learned</u>

Personal experiences often reveal common lessons. These stories offer valuable insights and advice that others can learn from and apply to their own lives. Find out what techniques have worked for others in managing their diabetes. These coping strategies can provide ideas and inspiration for your own journey.

Read messages of hope and perseverance. These stories provide encouragement and remind us that living well with diabetes is possible with the right mindset and effort.

Hear from a wide range of individuals, including children, teenagers, adults, and older adults. Each story offers a unique perspective on living with diabetes. Understand how diabetes management can vary across different cultures. These stories highlight the diverse ways people approach diabetes care based on cultural beliefs and practices. Learn from people who face additional challenges, such as other health conditions. Their stories show how they balance diabetes management with other medical needs. Many stories are available on social media and shared by diabetic help groups.

Advice for the Newly Diagnosed

<u>Tips for Adjusting to Life with Diabetes:</u>

Practical advice from those who have been newly diagnosed with diabetes can help you navigate the early stages of living with diabetes more smoothly.

<u>Support Systems:</u>

Discover the importance of finding and building a network of support. Learn how others have found support through family, friends, and community resources.

<u>Positive Outlook:</u>

Encouraging a proactive and optimistic approach to managing diabetes. These stories show how a positive outlook can make a significant difference in living well with the condition.

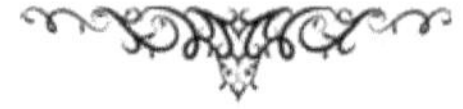

Chapter 17 - EXERCISE AND PHYSICAL ACTIVITY PLANS

Regular exercise and physical activity are vital components of managing diabetes and improving overall health. This chapter will guide you through creating effective and enjoyable exercise routines tailored to different fitness levels. We will discuss the many benefits of staying active, such as better blood sugar control, weight management, and enhanced mental well-being. You will find practical tips to stay motivated and safely incorporate physical activity into your daily life, whether through walking, yoga, strength training, or other activities. Emphasis will be placed on understanding your body's responses to exercise, preventing injuries, and recognizing when to seek medical advice. Empowering yourself with knowledge about exercise can significantly improve your quality of life and help you manage diabetes more effectively.

For individuals with diabetes, it is essential to engage in at least 150 minutes of exercise each week. The goal during these activities should be to reach 70% of their *Maximum*

Heart Rate (**MHR**), which varies based on age. To find the MHR, subtract your age from 220.

MHR = 220 – age of the person

For example, a 40-year-old should have an MHR of 180 beats per minute (220 minus 40). Therefore, this person should aim for a heart rate of 126 beats per minute (70% of 180) during exercise. This is referred to as the *Target Heart Rate* (**THR**).

Exercise Routines for Different Fitness Levels

Exercise is a powerful tool not only for managing diabetes but also for preventing its onset in individuals with prediabetes. The benefits of regular physical activity extend beyond weight loss, and consistency in exercise is key to achieving lasting results.

Beginner Level

<u>Walking</u>

No gym membership or costly equipment is needed to start walking. With a good pair of supportive shoes and a safe path, you can begin today. A 2021 review highlights that walking can help people with type 2 diabetes lower their blood pressure, HbA1c levels, and body mass index.

Begin with walking for about 10 to 15 minutes each day, and gradually increase the time to 30 minutes as you become more comfortable. Aim to walk at a brisk pace, which will help to increase your heart rate and improve your overall cardiovascular health.

<u>Basic Strength Training</u>

Start with simple bodyweight exercises such as squats, lunges, push-ups, and planks. These exercises do not require any special equipment and can be done at home. You can also use light weights or resistance bands to add a bit more challenge. Try to do these exercises 2 to 3 times a week, performing each exercise for 8 to 12 repetitions. For muscle strengthening, resistance bands are a versatile tool. To learn how to use them effectively, consult a professional trainer, attend a class, or follow workout videos. Resistance bands can also offer modest benefits for blood sugar management.

Calisthenics is an exercise method which uses your body weight to build strength. Common calisthenic exercises include push-ups, pull-ups, squats, lunges, and crunches. Aim to work every major muscle group in your body with body weight, weights, or resistance bands.

<u>Flexibility Exercises</u>

Incorporate stretching routines that focus on major muscle groups to improve flexibility. You might want to try beginner-level Yoga, Tai-chi or Pilates classes, or follow videos designed for beginners. Make stretching a part of your daily routine and hold each stretch for about 20 to 30 seconds to increase flexibility and prevent injuries.

A 2016 review indicates that yoga can aid in managing blood sugar, cholesterol levels, and weight, while also improving blood pressure, sleep quality, and mood. Consider joining a local yoga class to learn proper techniques and enhance your overall well-being.

Intermediate Level

<u>Cardio Workouts</u>

Increase your walking time to 45 to 60 minutes or add jogging or running to your routine for a more intense workout. You can also try cycling or swimming, aiming for about 30 to 45 minutes per session, 3 to 4 times a week. These activities will help improve your endurance and cardiovascular fitness. Participating in aerobic dance classes, such as Zumba, can help meet exercise goals. A 2015 study found that women with type 2 diabetes were more motivated to exercise and achieved better fitness and weight loss results after 16 weeks of Zumba.

Aquatic exercises, such as swimming, water aerobics, and aqua jogging, offer an excellent alternative for joint-friendly workouts. A 2017 review found that these activities can effectively lower blood sugar levels, much like land-based exercises. Many individuals with type 2 diabetes also suffer from arthritis, a condition that shares several risk factors with diabetes, including obesity. For those with joint pain, low-impact exercises like cycling can meet fitness goals while minimizing stress on the joints.

Strength Training

Move on to moderate weightlifting using dumbbells, kettlebells, or gym machines. Focus on full-body workouts, doing exercises 3 to 4 times a week with 10 to 15 repetitions per exercise. Concentrate on compound movements like deadlifts, bench presses, and rows, which work multiple muscle groups at once. Strength training builds muscle mass, which boosts daily calorie burn and improves blood sugar control. Incorporate weightlifting into your routine using machines, free weights, or even household items like canned goods or water bottles.

Flexibility and Balance

Engage in intermediate Yoga or Pilates classes to further enhance your flexibility and balance. You can also perform balance exercises, such as single leg stands or stability ball exercises. Aim to practice these 2 to 3 times a week to build strength and coordination.

Advanced Level

Intense Cardio Exercise

For a more challenging cardio workout, try *High-Intensity Interval Training* (**HIIT**). This involves doing short bursts of very intense activity followed by periods of rest. You can also incorporate sprints or hill running into your routine. Aim for 30 to 45 minutes of intense cardio 4 to 5 times a week to boost your fitness level.

Struggling to stay motivated? Joining a recreational sports team may help. The social interaction and commitment to teammates can provide the motivation needed for regular exercise. Consider sports like basketball, soccer, softball, pairs tennis, or ultimate frisbee for a solid aerobic workout.

Advanced Strength Training

Advanced strength training includes heavy weightlifting exercises such as squats, deadlifts, bench presses, and pull-ups. You might follow split routines where you focus on different muscle groups on different days. Train 4 to 5 times a week with 6 to 10 repetitions per exercise to increase muscle strength and mass.

Advanced Flexibility and Balance

Participate in advanced Yoga or Pilates sessions to enhance your flexibility and balance further. Incorporate dynamic stretches, such as leg swings, arm circles, and hip rotations, into your routine. Aim to practice these daily or include them as part of your warm-up and cool-down routines to maintain overall flexibility and balance.

Tips for Staying Motivated

<u>Set Clear Goals</u>

Establish both short-term goals, such as losing a few pounds or improving your fitness level in a few weeks, and long-term goals, like preparing for a specific event or reaching a significant milestone in your fitness journey. Setting clear goals helps you stay focused and motivated.

Make sure your goals follow the SMART criteria, which stands for Specific, Measurable, Achievable, Relevant, and Time-bound. This means your goals should be clearly defined, you should be able to measure your progress, they should be realistic and relevant to your life, and you should set a timeframe for achieving them.

<u>Track Progress</u>

Write down details of your workouts in an exercise journal. Record how long you exercised, the intensity of the workout, and how you felt afterward. This can help you see your progress over time and keep you motivated to continue.

Consider using fitness apps or wearables that track your steps, heart rate, and calories burned. These tools can provide valuable insights into your activity levels and help you stay on track with your fitness goals.

<u>Find Enjoyable Activities</u>

Try out various types of physical activities to find what you enjoy the most. Whether it is dancing, martial arts, or playing sports, engaging in exercises that you find fun will make it easier to stick with them.

Participate in group fitness classes or join local sports teams. Activities like Yoga, Zumba, or cycling groups not only offer structured workouts but also provide a sense of community and social interaction, which can enhance your motivation.

Create a Routine

Set a specific time each day or week for your workouts and stick to it. By making exercise a regular part of your schedule, you create a routine that becomes a natural and expected part of your day.

Consider your workout sessions as important appointments that you cannot miss. Treating them as non-negotiable parts of your day helps ensure that you consistently make time for physical activity.

Social Support

Working out with friends or family members can make exercise more enjoyable and provide a sense of accountability. Having a workout buddy can also make the experience more fun and motivating.

Engage with fitness communities online or in person. Participate in online forums, local fitness clubs, or social media groups dedicated to fitness. Being part of a community can offer support, encouragement, and additional motivation.

Reward Yourself

Establish milestones for your fitness journey and reward yourself when you reach them. Choose non-food rewards such as new workout gear, a relaxing spa day, or other treats that celebrate your hard work and progress.

Acknowledge and celebrate your achievements, no matter how small. Recognizing your progress helps maintain motivation and reinforces the positive behavior you are striving for.

<u>Stay Inspired</u>

Follow fitness influencers on social media, blogs, or YouTube channels to stay inspired. Their posts, videos, and tips can provide motivation and new ideas for your workouts.

Read books, articles, or testimonials from individuals who have achieved fitness goals or overcome challenges. Learning about other people's success stories can inspire you and give you ideas for your own journey.

<u>Overcome Obstacles</u>

Prepare for potential setbacks such as bad weather, busy days, or minor injuries. Having backup plans, like indoor workout options or alternative exercise routines, can help you stay on track despite these challenges.

Even if you cannot complete a full workout, doing a shorter session is better than skipping exercise altogether. Staying consistent, even with shorter or less intense workouts, helps you maintain your routine and progress over time.

Safety Considerations

<u>Consult Healthcare Providers</u>

Before starting any new exercise routine, it is important to talk to your doctor, especially if you are 30 or older. This ensures that the exercise you plan to do is suitable and safe for your health condition. Your doctor can help you determine what types of exercises are appropriate and if there are any specific precautions you need to take. Your doctor may plan a *Treadmill Exercise Test* (**TMT**) to assess your exercise capacity before permitting you to undertake strenuous exercise. The elderly are advised to exercise at the beginner level or the intermediate level if their fitness permits. Advanced level of exercise may not suit them.

If you have any medical conditions or take medications (other than for diabetes), your exercise plan might need to be adjusted. Those with complications like Retinopathy, High Blood Pressure and Cardiac problems should plan their exercise on the advice of their doctors only. Getting personalized advice from your healthcare provider helps to tailor your exercise routine to your individual needs, ensuring you stay safe while achieving your fitness goals. It is ideal to have a bracelet or a dog tag showing that you are diabetic. This

> *Samuel, a 50-year-old businessman, was recently diagnosed with type 2 diabetes. His lifestyle, marked by long hours of sedentary work and poor eating habits, had led to significant weight gain and high cholesterol levels. Samuel's father had also been diabetic and tragically passed away at the age of 55 from a heart attack, a fact that weighed heavily on Samuel as he received his diagnosis.*
>
> *Understanding the gravity of the situation, Samuel's physician prescribed a weight-reducing diabetic diet, crafted by a dietitian, along with medications to control both his blood sugar and cholesterol levels. Recognizing Samuel's increased risk for heart disease, the doctor emphasized the importance of regular exercise. However, before starting any physical activity, Samuel underwent a Treadmill Exercise Test to ensure his heart could handle the strain. When Samuel successfully reached his Target Heart Rate of 119 beats per minute, without any adverse symptoms, the doctor recommended brisk walking and swimming as safe and effective exercises.*
>
> *Over the next three months, Samuel adhered strictly to his new lifestyle. His efforts paid off — he lost weight, his blood sugar and cholesterol levels stabilized, and he experienced a renewed sense of physical and mental well-being. Samuel's commitment to his health not only improved his condition but also gave him the confidence to continue managing his diabetes effectively.*

will help others in the event there is any mishap. In the event of any symptoms like chest pain, dizziness or breathlessness, the exercise should be terminated.

<u>Monitor Blood Glucose Levels</u>

To prevent issues like low or high blood sugar, it is important to monitor your blood glucose levels regularly. Check them before you start exercising, during the activity if needed, and after you finish. This helps in managing your blood sugar effectively and avoiding potential complications. Always have fast-acting carbohydrates with you during exercise, such as glucose tablets, juice, or snacks in the event of blood sugar becoming low during exertion. These can quickly raise your blood sugar levels if you experience hypoglycemia, ensuring you have a way to manage your levels on the spot.

<u>Warm-Up and Cool-Down</u>

Always begin your exercise session with 5-10 minutes of light cardio, like brisk walking or jogging, combined with dynamic stretches. This 'warm up' helps prepare your muscles and joints for the workout, reducing the risk of injury.

After exercising, spend 5-10 minutes doing gentle stretching and deep breathing exercises. This 'cool down' helps your body transition back to a resting state, reduces muscle soreness, and promotes overall recovery.

<u>Stay Hydrated</u>

Make sure to drink water before, during, and after your workout to stay hydrated. Proper hydration helps your body function effectively and prevents dehydration, which can affect your performance and health.

Unless you specifically need them to manage blood sugar levels, it is best to avoid sugary sports drinks. Opt for water instead to stay hydrated and keep your sugar intake in check.

<u>Proper Footwear and Equipment</u>

Choose shoes that provide good support and cushioning to prevent foot injuries. Proper footwear is crucial in avoiding problems such as blisters, calluses, and other foot issues, especially during high-impact activities.

Make sure to use the right equipment for your exercises, such as weights, mats, or resistance bands. Using the proper gear helps ensure that you perform exercises correctly and safely, reducing the risk of injury. Get professional advice from a trainer when needed.

<u>Recognize Warning Signs</u>

Be aware of signs of low blood sugar, which include dizziness, shaking, sweating, and confusion. If you experience these symptoms, stop exercising and take action to raise your blood sugar levels.

Symptoms of high blood sugar include excessive thirst, frequent urination, and fatigue. If you notice these signs, it is important to address them promptly and consider adjusting your exercise or checking your blood sugar levels.

If you experience severe symptoms such as chest pain or severe shortness of breath, stop exercising immediately and seek medical help. These could be signs of a serious health issue that needs attention.

<u>Adapt Exercises as Needed</u>

Adjust the intensity of your workouts based on your current fitness level, health status, and blood glucose levels. Tailoring your exercise routine helps you manage your health effectively while still getting the benefits of physical activity.

Consider low-impact exercises like swimming, cycling, or walking. These activities are easier on the joints and can be a good choice if you need to protect your joints or have certain health concerns. The elderly should not do vigorous exercises and avoid those where the risk of fall is possible.

<u>Listen to Your Body</u>

It is important to rest when your body needs it to prevent overtraining and injury. Pay attention to signs of fatigue or discomfort and take breaks as necessary to allow your body to recover.

Differentiate between normal exercise discomfort and potential injury. If you experience pain that feels more than just muscle soreness, it is important to stop and assess whether you might be at risk of an injury.

These safety considerations are crucial for ensuring that your exercise routine is both effective and safe. By consulting with healthcare providers, monitoring your blood glucose levels, staying hydrated, and using proper equipment, you can enjoy a productive and safe exercise experience.

<u>Benefits of Exercise.</u>

Exercise has many benefits.

- o It helps the pancreas work better and makes the body more responsive to insulin.
- o Exercise also boosts memory and can prevent or delay heart problems.
- o For women, staying active before pregnancy lowers the risk of developing diabetes during pregnancy – GDM.
- o Additionally, exercise aids in weight control, balance and strengthens muscles and bones. This is particularly important for older adults, as it significantly reduces the risk of falls.

o Hormones released during exercise contribute to a feeling of well-being.

o Exercise is well-known for its numerous physical health benefits, but it also has significant positive effects on mental health and overall well-being. One of the reasons for this is the release of certain hormones during exercise.

Learn the benefits of exercising. Here are the key hormones that are released during physical activity and contribute to a feeling of well-being:

<u>Endorphins</u> are often referred to as the body's natural painkillers. They are neurotransmitters produced by the brain and nervous system that can help reduce pain and stress. They are known to create a feeling of euphoria, often termed as the *"runner's high."* This euphoric feeling helps reduce stress and anxiety, leaving individuals feeling more relaxed and happier after exercise.

<u>Dopamine</u> is a neurotransmitter that plays a crucial role in the reward and pleasure centers of the brain. It is associated with feelings of enjoyment and reinforcement to continue engaging in pleasurable activities. During exercise, dopamine levels increase, leading to improved mood and a sense of accomplishment and motivation.

<u>Serotonin</u> is a neurotransmitter that helps regulate mood, appetite, and sleep. It is often called the *"feel-good"* hormone because of its strong impact on mood and overall sense of well-being. Exercise boosts serotonin levels, which can help alleviate feelings of depression and anxiety, promoting a positive mood and better mental health.

<u>Norepinephrine</u> is both a hormone and a neurotransmitter. It is involved in the body's fight or flight response and helps increase alertness, arousal, and attention. Exercise increases norepinephrine levels, enhancing mood,

focus, and energy levels, which contributes to a sense of mental clarity and well-being.

Adrenaline (Epinephrine) is a hormone released by the adrenal glands in response to stress and exercise. It prepares the body for physical exertion by increasing heart rate, blood flow to muscles, and energy availability. The surge of adrenaline during exercise can lead to heightened alertness and a feeling of increased vitality and excitement.

Brain-Derived Neurotrophic Factor (**BDNF**) is a protein that supports the survival of existing neurons and encourages the growth of new neurons and synapses. It is crucial for long-term memory, learning, and overall cognitive function. Exercise boosts BDNF levels, which can improve brain function and mental clarity, contributing to a sense of well-being and cognitive sharpness.

Endocannabinoids are neurotransmitters that bind to certain receptors in the brain. They play a role in regulating mood, pain sensation, appetite, and memory. Exercise increases the production of endocannabinoids, which can enhance mood, reduce pain, and promote relaxation, leading to an overall feeling of well-being.

The release of these hormones and neurotransmitters during exercise not only enhances physical health but also significantly boosts mental and emotional well-being. Thus, regular physical activity can lead to sustained improvements in mood, reduced stress and anxiety, and an overall enhanced quality of life.

Chapter 18 - NUTRITIONAL RECIPES AND MEAL PLANS

Managing diabetes effectively requires careful attention to diet. This chapter focuses on the importance of planning and portioning meals to maintain stable blood sugar levels. Working with a dietitian can help create a personalized meal plan that meets individual needs and preferences. It is essential to understand that meal plans vary from person to person and can be influenced by cultural factors. For example, a meal plan suitable for someone in the United States may differ significantly from one designed for someone in India. In this chapter, you will find sample meal plans from both Western and Eastern (Indian) cuisines, offering practical examples to help you manage your diabetes through diet. Proper meal planning and portion control can play a vital role in your overall diabetes management and improve your quality of life. Both vegetarian and non-vegetarian recipes are mentioned.

A vegetarian diet reduces the risk of diabetes and improves the blood glucose levels in those having the disease.

It has been shown that the mean body mass index is lowest in Vegans (no dairy), a bit higher in Vegetarians and highest in Non-vegetarians. The prevalence of diabetes is also lowest in vegans and highest in non-vegetarians.

Some terms are worth noting in relation to diet in diabetes. A **Serving** size means the specific amount of food defined as standard measurements like cup, ounce or piece. A ***Portion*** is the amount of food put on the plate. **An Exchange** is one serving within a group – e.g. Carbohydrate or one starch exchange = 3 oz baked potato *or* ½ cup corn *or* 1/3 cup baked beans.

SOME EASY AND HEALTHY RECIPES FOR DIABETICS

Breakfast Recipes

Oatmeal with Berries and Nuts

Ingredients: Rolled oats, fresh berries, nuts (such as almonds or walnuts), and cinnamon.

Preparation: Begin by cooking the rolled oats according to the package instructions. Once the oats are cooked, add a generous serving of fresh berries on top. Sprinkle a handful of nuts and a dash of cinnamon to finish.

Nutritional Benefits: This breakfast is beneficial because it has a low glycemic index, meaning it will not spike your blood sugar levels. It is also rich in fiber, which aids digestion, and contains heart-healthy fats from the nuts.

Veggie Omelette

Ingredients: Eggs or egg whites, fresh spinach, chopped tomatoes, bell peppers, onions, and a small amount of low-fat cheese.

Preparation: Start by whisking the eggs or egg whites in a bowl. Pour the eggs into a heated, non-stick skillet. Once they start to set, add the spinach, tomatoes, bell peppers, and onions. Cook until the vegetables are tender, and the eggs are fully cooked. Sprinkle some low-fat cheese on top before folding the omelette.

Nutritional Benefits: This meal is packed with protein, which is essential for muscle maintenance. It is low in carbohydrates, making it great for managing blood sugar levels, and it is full of vitamins from the vegetables.

Lunch Recipes

Quinoa Salad with Grilled Chicken

Ingredients: Quinoa, grilled chicken breast, mixed greens, cherry tomatoes, cucumbers, olive oil, and lemon juice.

Preparation: Cook the quinoa as directed on the package. While the quinoa is cooking, grill the chicken breast until it is fully cooked. Once both are ready, toss them together with mixed greens, halved cherry tomatoes, and sliced cucumbers. Dress with a mixture of olive oil and lemon juice.

Nutritional Benefits: This salad is high in protein, which helps keep you full and satisfied. It is also rich in fiber and contains a variety of essential nutrients from vegetables and quinoa.

Lentil Soup

Ingredients: Lentils, chopped carrots, celery, onions, garlic, vegetable broth, and your favorite spices.

Preparation: Begin by sautéing the onions, garlic, carrots, and celery in a large pot until they are soft. Add the lentils and vegetable broth, then bring the mixture to a boil. Reduce the heat and let it simmer until the lentils are tender. Season with spices to taste.

Nutritional Benefits: This soup is an excellent source of plant-based protein and fiber, which help maintain steady blood sugar levels. It is also low in fat, making it a heart-healthy option.

Dinner Recipes

Baked Salmon with Asparagus

Ingredients: Salmon fillets, fresh asparagus, olive oil, lemon, herbs (such as dill or parsley), and garlic.

Preparation: Preheat your oven to 375°F (190°C). Place the salmon fillets and asparagus on a baking sheet. Drizzle them with olive oil and lemon juice, then sprinkle with herbs and minced garlic. Bake for about 20 minutes or until the salmon is cooked through and the asparagus is tender.

Nutritional Benefits: Salmon is rich in omega-3 fatty acids, which are good for heart health. This meal is also a great source of lean protein and is low in carbohydrates, making it ideal for managing diabetes.

Stuffed Bell Peppers

Ingredients: Bell peppers, lean ground turkey or beef, cooked brown rice, diced tomatoes, chopped onions, and your favorite spices.

Preparation: Preheat your oven to 375°F (190°C). Cut the tops off the bell peppers and remove the seeds. In a skillet, cook the ground meat with onions and spices until fully cooked. Mix in the cooked brown rice and diced tomatoes. Stuff the bell peppers with the mixture and place them in a baking dish. Bake for about 30 minutes or until the peppers are tender.

Nutritional Benefits: This meal provides a balance of protein, fiber, and vitamins, making it a nutritious choice. The combination of lean meat and brown rice helps manage blood sugar levels effectively.

Snack Recipes

Greek Yogurt with Nuts and Seeds

Ingredients: Plain Greek yogurt, mixed nuts (such as almonds and walnuts), chia seeds, and flaxseeds.

Preparation: Scoop the Greek yogurt into a bowl. Top it with a handful of mixed nuts and a sprinkle of chia and flaxseeds. Stir to combine and enjoy.

Nutritional Benefits: Greek yogurt is high in protein, which helps keep you full. The nuts and seeds add healthy fats and fiber, making this a well-rounded and satisfying snack.

Veggie Sticks with Hummus

Ingredients: Carrot sticks, celery sticks, bell pepper strips, and hummus.

Preparation: Slice the vegetables into sticks or strips. Serve with a side of hummus for dipping.

Nutritional Benefits: This snack is rich in fiber, low in calories, and packed with nutrients. The hummus provides a good source of protein and healthy fats.

Dessert Recipes

Chia Seed Pudding

Ingredients: Chia seeds, almond milk, vanilla extract, and fresh berries.

Preparation: In a bowl, mix the chia seeds with almond milk and a splash of vanilla extract. Stir well and let it sit in the refrigerator for at least an hour, or until it thickens to a pudding-like consistency. Top with fresh berries before serving.

Nutritional Benefits: Chia seeds are high in fiber and omega-3 fatty acids, which are good for heart health. This dessert is also low in sugar, making it a healthy option for managing diabetes.

Baked Apples with Cinnamon

Ingredients: Apples, cinnamon, nutmeg, and a small amount of honey or sugar substitute.

Preparation: Preheat your oven to 350°F (175°C). Core the apples and place them in a baking dish. Sprinkle cinnamon and nutmeg and drizzle a small amount of honey or sugar substitute over them. Bake for about 20-30 minutes or until the apples are tender.

Nutritional Benefits: Baked apples are naturally sweet and packed with vitamins and antioxidants. This dessert is a healthy way to satisfy your sweet tooth without adding too much sugar.

Sample Meal Plans

One-Day Meal Plan

Breakfast: Start your day with a bowl of Greek yogurt topped with a mix of crunchy nuts and sweet berries. This breakfast is quick to prepare and provides a good balance of protein and antioxidants to kickstart your morning.

Snack: For a mid-morning snack, enjoy a selection of fresh veggie sticks like carrots, celery, and bell peppers, paired with a creamy hummus dip. This snack is both satisfying and nutritious, offering fiber and essential vitamins.

Lunch: For lunch, have a hearty quinoa salad mixed with grilled chicken breast, fresh greens, cherry tomatoes, and cucumbers, all drizzled with a simple olive oil and lemon dressing. This meal is filling and packed with protein and healthy fats.

Snack: In the afternoon, have some crisp apple slices dipped in smooth almond butter. This snack combines the natural sweetness of the apple with the creamy richness of almond butter, providing a balanced and tasty treat.

Dinner: For dinner, enjoy a piece of baked salmon served with a side of tender asparagus. This meal is easy to prepare and offers a great source of omega-3 fatty acids and lean protein.

Dessert: End your day with a delicious chia seed pudding made by soaking chia seeds in almond milk, flavored with a touch of vanilla, and topped with fresh berries. This dessert is not only tasty but also high in fiber and healthy fats.

Weekly Meal Plan

Monday

Breakfast: Start your week with a warm bowl of oatmeal topped with fresh berries and crunchy nuts. This combination is filling and provides a good amount of fiber and healthy fats.

Lunch: For lunch, enjoy a comforting bowl of lentil soup, packed with vegetables like carrots, celery, and onions. This soup is nutritious and perfect for a cozy midday meal.

Dinner: Finish the day with stuffed bell peppers filled with a mixture of lean ground turkey or beef, brown rice, and diced tomatoes. This dish is hearty and balanced, offering plenty of protein and fiber.

Tuesday

Breakfast: Whip up a veggie omelette using eggs or egg whites, packed with fresh spinach, tomatoes, bell peppers, and onions. This breakfast is high in protein and vitamins.

Lunch: Have a quinoa salad with grilled chicken, mixed greens, cherry tomatoes, and cucumbers for lunch. This salad is both refreshing and satisfying.

Dinner: For dinner, enjoy baked salmon served with a side of roasted asparagus. This meal is rich in omega-3 fatty acids and lean protein, making it a healthy choice.

Wednesday

Breakfast: Start the day with a bowl of Greek yogurt topped with a mix of nuts and seeds. This breakfast is high in protein and healthy fats.

Lunch: For lunch, have a spinach and chicken salad, which is light yet packed with nutrients and protein.

Dinner: Enjoy a dinner of grilled tofu served with mixed vegetables. This meal is a great source of plant-based protein and vitamins.

Thursday

Breakfast: Blend up a smoothie with fresh spinach, creamy avocado, and a scoop of protein powder for a nutritious and energizing breakfast.

Lunch: Enjoy a turkey and avocado wrap for lunch. This meal is easy to make and offers a good balance of protein and healthy fats.

Dinner: Have roasted chicken with a side of Brussels sprouts for dinner. This meal is rich in protein and fiber, making it a wholesome choice.

Friday

Breakfast: Start your day with whole grain toast topped with mashed avocado and a poached egg. This breakfast is filling and offers healthy fats and protein.

Lunch: For lunch, have a hearty lentil and vegetable stew. This meal is packed with fiber and plant-based protein.

Dinner: Enjoy grilled shrimp served with quinoa and a mix of colorful vegetables for dinner. This meal is light yet satisfying, offering a good mix of protein and nutrients.

Saturday

Breakfast: Have a bowl of chia seed pudding topped with fresh berries for breakfast. This meal is rich in fiber and healthy fats.

Lunch: For lunch, enjoy a mixed green salad topped with a variety of nuts and seeds. This salad is light, nutritious, and packed with healthy fats and fiber.

Dinner: End the day with stuffed bell peppers filled with a mixture of lean meat, brown rice, and vegetables. This dish is hearty and balanced, providing plenty of protein and fiber.

Sunday

Breakfast: Start your Sunday with a smoothie bowl topped with fresh fruits and a sprinkle of nuts. This breakfast is refreshing and packed with vitamins and healthy fats.

Lunch: For lunch, have a quinoa and black bean salad, which is high in protein and fiber.

Dinner: Finish the week with baked fish served with a side of steamed broccoli and sweet potatoes. This meal is nutritious and balanced, offering lean protein and essential vitamins.

This detailed outline should provide a comprehensive framework for discussing easy and healthy recipes for diabetics, including breakfast, lunch, dinner, snacks, and desserts, as well as sample meal plans for both a single day and an entire week. This is given only as a suggestion. Readers are encouraged to experiment with newer recipes with ingredients of their choice and design their own recipes. More recipes can be obtained from books dedicated to diabetic recipes for different cultures and tastes. These recipes given above were derived from the internet. Readers are advised to read books on recipes for diabetics published by various authors, chefs and gourmets to get more information. [See chapter 20 on *Resources and Support*].

The Mediterranean Diet: A Path to Long-Term Health.

The Mediterranean diet, hailed as one of the healthiest diets in the world, offers a sustainable approach to weight loss and overall well-being. Rooted in the dietary habits of countries bordering the Mediterranean Sea, this diet is more of a lifestyle choice, emphasizing the enjoyment of meals with others and the consumption of fresh, wholesome foods.

<u>The Mediterranean Diet Pyramid</u> (**Fig 1**)

- At the base of the Mediterranean Diet Pyramid is the importance of enjoying meals in the company of others, promoting social interaction and mindful eating.
- Moving up the pyramid, the next level includes an abundance of fruits, vegetables, whole grains, olive oil, beans, nuts, legumes, seeds, herbs, and spices. These plant-based foods form the cornerstone of the diet, providing essential nutrients and antioxidants.
- Fish and seafood are recommended at least twice a week, offering a rich source of omega-3 fatty acids, which are beneficial for heart health.
- Poultry, eggs, cheese, and yogurt are included in moderation, providing necessary protein and calcium.

- At the top of the pyramid are meats and sweets, which should be consumed less often.

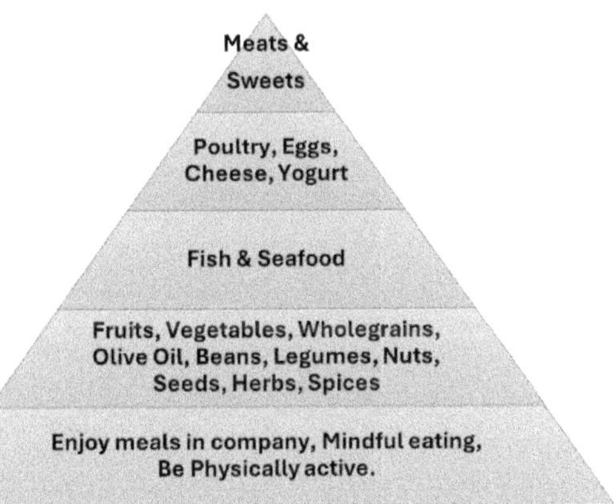

Fig. 1 Shows the foods included in Mediterranean Diet

<u>Key Principles and Benefits</u>

Water is the primary beverage, with wine allowed in moderation—up to 5 ounces daily for those over 65, and 10 ounces for younger adults. The Mediterranean diet has numerous health benefits attributed to it:

- By emphasizing whole foods and healthy fats, this diet helps in maintaining stable blood sugar levels.

- It reduces the risk of strokes and heart attacks.

- Improved mental capacity and potential reversal of symptoms of Parkinson's and Alzheimer's diseases.

- A diet rich in antioxidants and anti-inflammatory foods contributes to a longer life.

- Reduced risk of cancer due to a high intake of fruits, vegetables, and whole grains.

Mediterranean diet emphasizes the following:

- Plant-Based Foods with focus on fruits, vegetables, whole grains, legumes, and nuts instead of meat.

- Local Produce which bases meals around fresh, local produce ensures higher nutrient intake rather than packaged foods.

- Using extra virgin olive oil as the primary fat source instead of saturated fats like butter.

- Fresh Herbs and Spices are used in flavoring foods instead of salt.

- Consuming fresh fish two or three times a week.

- Limiting red meat and sweets to special occasions.

- Including poultry and dairy products two or three times a week.

The Mediterranean diet encourages communal eating, physical activity, and a balanced approach to food, making it not just a diet, but a lifestyle that supports long-term health and weight management.

Some Randon Tips for Diabetics for Eating Out and Special Occasions

<u>Choosing Restaurants</u>

When selecting a restaurant, look for places that offer healthy menu options. Aim for restaurants that have a variety of salads, grilled meats, and whole grain dishes. These types of meals are generally lower in unhealthy fats and added sugars.

It is also a good idea to check out the restaurant's menu online before you go. This way, you can identify which dishes are better for managing diabetes and plan your meal in advance. Knowing what you can order ahead of time can help you make healthier choices and avoid being tempted by less nutritious options once you are there.

<u>Making Healthier Choices</u>

When dining out, pay attention to portion sizes. To avoid overeating, consider asking for half portions of dishes or sharing a meal with someone else. This way, you can enjoy the flavors without consuming too many calories or carbs.

Customize your meal to make it healthier. You can ask for steamed vegetables instead of fried ones, request that your food be grilled instead of fried, and ask for dressings and sauces on the side so you can control how much you use. These small adjustments can make a big difference to the overall healthiness of your meal.

Some low Glycemic Index (GI) fruits are Apricots, Cherries, Grapefruit, Pears, Apples, Oranges, Plums, Strawberries, Peach and Grapes.

Some High Sugary fruits that one should be vary of are Dried fruits, Canned fruits with added sugar, Fruit juices, Lychee, Pineapple, Papaya. These have a high GI.

Try to limit foods that are high in carbohydrates and sugars. For example, avoid bread baskets, sugary drinks, and rich desserts that can cause your blood sugar to spike. Opt for water or unsweetened beverages and choose fresh fruit or a small serving of a healthier dessert option if you're craving something sweet.

<u>Managing Special Occasions</u>

For special events or gatherings, plan ahead to help manage your food intake. Eating a small, healthy snack before you go for a party can help you avoid arriving too hungry and overeating when you get there. Choose snacks that are high in protein or fiber to keep you satisfied.

At the event, try to fill your plate with lean proteins and plenty of vegetables. Lean meats, like chicken or fish, and a variety of colorful vegetables will help keep your meal balanced and nutritious.

If you plan to have an alcoholic drink, be mindful of your choices. Choose low-carb options like dry wine or spirits mixed with water or diet soda, rather than sugary cocktails. This will help you manage your blood sugar levels while still enjoying the occasion.

The GI of some cereals are - Cornflakes – 79, Muesli – 57, Oatmeal – 55, Wheat bran cereals – 45.

Some bedtime routines for diabetics

A few suggestions for bedtime routine to follow are:

- ✓ Check blood sugar before bedtime. If found low, one should take a bedtime snack.
- ✓ Avoid caffeine a few hours before bedtime.
- ✓ Limit alcohol intake in the evening and night.
- ✓ Walk for 15-20 minutes after dinner before going to bed. But do not do vigorous exercise.
- ✓ The bedroom should be quiet, dimly lit with a temperature around 16-20°C [60 - 67°F].
- ✓ A warm shower before bedtime promotes good sleep.
- ✓ Do not watch TV or the mobile phone for an hour prior to bedtime. Light reading helps.
- ✓ Having high carbs at night or insufficient medication can cause a rise of blood glucose around 3 – 8 am. This is called the '*Dawn Phenomenon*.'

Holiday Meals

During the holidays, balance is key. Allow yourself to enjoy small portions of your favorite holiday dishes but keep moderation in mind. It is okay to indulge a little but try to do so in a way that does not negatively impact your blood sugar control.

You can also prepare and bring a diabetes-friendly dish to share with others. This way, you ensure that there will be a healthy option available that fits your dietary needs.

Incorporate physical activity into your holiday routines. Whether it is a walk after a meal or playing an active game with family, staying active can help balance out any extra calories you might consume.

Some good snacks for Diabetics

Some snacks which the people with diabetes can take in between meals to maintain a uniform blood glucose are - Yogurt, Berries, Hardboiled egg, Almonds, Vegetable salad with hummus, Avocado, Apple, Beef sticks, Roasted chickpeas, Cottage cheese, Crackers, Tuna Salad, Popcorn, Energy bites and Protein bars.

Healthy Natural Sweeteners

Some people need a sweetener with their coffee or tea. Healthy sweeteners are naturally occurring ones which may be used. Some of these are Stevia (*Methi Tulsi*), Erythritol, Xylitol, Monk fruit sweetener and Yacon syrup. Some of these may cause digestive problems like bloating and hence, it is better to use them sparingly.

Artificial sweeteners like Sucralose, Aspartame, Saccharin, Neotame, Acesulfame potassium are also useful. They may leave an after taste which many do not like. Some of these are mentioned as detrimental to health and hence it is best to use them sparingly.

Travel Tips

When traveling, pack a variety of healthy snacks to keep you on track with your eating plan. Good options include nuts, seeds, fresh fruits, and whole grain crackers. These snacks are easy to carry and will help you avoid unhealthy choices when you are on the go.

Staying hydrated is also important. Drink plenty of water throughout your trip and try to avoid sugary drinks that can affect your blood sugar levels.

Keep your routine as consistent as possible. Stick to your regular mealtimes and remember to monitor your blood glucose levels as needed. This will help you stay on top of your diabetes management, even when you are away from home.

SOUTH INDIAN VEGETARIAN RECIPES

Here are some recipes for diabetic patients while keeping the traditional South Indian Vegetarian flavors:

Breakfast

<u>Vegetable Upma</u>

Ingredients: Semolina (rava) made from whole grain or semolina with added fiber, mixed vegetables (carrots, peas, beans), mustard seeds, curry leaves, green chilies, urad dal (black gram), chana dal (split chickpeas), turmeric, roasted cashew nuts and salt.

Preparation: Roast the whole grain semolina until lightly golden. In a pan, heat a small amount of oil and add mustard seeds, urad dal, and chana dal. Once they splutter, add chopped vegetables, green chilies, and curry leaves. Add turmeric and salt. Stir in the semolina and cook with water until the mixture is thick and cooked through. May be garnished with roasted cashew nuts.

Note: Use more vegetables and less semolina to keep the carbohydrate content lower.

Snack 1

Curd Rice

Ingredients: Cooked brown rice or a mix of brown rice and cauliflower rice (finely chopped cauliflower), plain yogurt (curd) - low-fat or unsweetened, mustard seeds, curry leaves, green chilies, ginger, coriander leaves, and salt.

Preparation: Mix plain yogurt with cooked brown rice or cauliflower rice. In a separate pan, heat a small amount of oil, add mustard seeds, chopped green chilies, and curry leaves. Fry briefly and pour over the rice and yogurt mixture. Garnish with chopped coriander leaves.

Note: Cauliflower rice can be used to reduce the carbohydrate content of the meal.

Lunch

Sambar with Rice

Ingredients: Toor dal (pigeon peas), mixed vegetables (drumstick, carrots, beans, Okra), tamarind, sambar powder, mustard seeds, curry leaves, dried red chilies, and salt.

Preparation: Cook Toor dal and vegetables in a pressure cooker. Add tamarind extract and sambar powder. Simmer until flavors blend. In a separate pan, prepare a tempering with mustard seeds, curry leaves, and dried red chilies, then add to the sambar. Serve with a small portion of steamed brown rice or cauliflower rice.

Note: Use less rice and more vegetables to control carbohydrate intake.

Coconut Chutney

Ingredients: Fresh coconut (grated), green chilies, ginger, tamarind, mustard seeds, curry leaves, and salt.

Preparation: Blend grated coconut with green chilies, ginger, and a small amount of tamarind into a smooth paste. Heat a small amount of oil, add mustard seeds and curry leaves for tempering, and pour over the chutney.

Note: Use minimal coconut and focus on other ingredients to keep the fat content lower.

Snack 2

Fruit Salad

Ingredients: Seasonal fruits like apples, bananas, oranges, and a small amount of pomegranate, with a dash of lemon juice.

Preparation: Chop fruits into bite-sized pieces. Toss with a bit of lemon juice to prevent browning and enhance flavor.

Note: Choose fruits with a lower glycemic index, like apples and berries, and avoid high-sugar fruits like bananas in excess.

Dinner

Vegetable Biryani

Ingredients: Basmati rice (use in moderation), mixed vegetables (potatoes, carrots, peas), biryani spices (cloves, cinnamon, cardamom), yogurt (low-fat or unsweetened), chopped onions, ginger-garlic paste, and salt.

Preparation: Sauté onions, ginger-garlic paste, and spices in a small amount of oil. Add vegetables and cook until partially tender. Mix in yogurt and add a small amount of basmati rice with water. Cook until rice and vegetables are done.

Note: Use less rice and more vegetables and opt for cauliflower rice or brown rice if preferred.

Raita

Ingredients: Plain yogurt (low-fat or unsweetened), cucumber, cumin powder, coriander leaves, and salt.

Preparation: Grate or finely chop cucumber and mix with yogurt. Add cumin powder and salt. Garnish with chopped coriander leaves.

Note: Opt for low-fat or unsweetened yogurt to reduce calorie and sugar intake.

This revised meal plan retains the traditional South Indian flavors while being more mindful of carbohydrate content and using ingredients that are better suited for managing blood sugar levels.

A modified version of a sample meal plan that is suitable for diabetics is given below. It emphasizes low glycemic index foods, balanced portions, and good sources of fiber and protein for Vegetarians from South India. Five meal exchanges are also given below

Diabetic-Friendly South Indian Vegetarian Meal Plan

Breakfast

Moong Dal Chilla (Savory Pancakes)

Ingredients: Moong dal (yellow split gram), green chilies, ginger, curry leaves, chopped vegetables (carrot, spinach), and a small amount of cumin.

Preparation: Soak moong dal overnight, blend into a batter with vegetables and spices, and cook the pancakes on a non-stick pan.

Nutritional Benefits: High in protein and fiber, low in glycemic index.

Low-Fat Curd (Yogurt)

Ingredients: Plain low-fat curd, with a few mint leaves for flavor.

Preparation: Serve chilled or at room temperature.

Nutritional Benefits: Provides probiotics and calcium without added sugars.

Snack 1

Raw Vegetable Sticks with Mint Chutney

Ingredients: Carrot sticks, cucumber sticks, and a small serving of mint chutney made from mint leaves, cilantro, and a small amount of lemon juice ground into a paste.

Preparation: Slice vegetables and serve with chutney.

Nutritional Benefits: Low in calories, high in fiber, and helps in keeping blood sugar levels steady.

Lunch

Brown Rice and Mixed Vegetable Sambar

Ingredients: Brown rice, mixed vegetables (like drumsticks, carrots, beans), Toor dal (pigeon peas), tamarind, and sambar spices.

Preparation: Cook brown rice and prepare sambar by cooking Toor dal with vegetables and spices.

Nutritional Benefits: Brown rice is lower in glycemic index compared to white rice, and sambar provides fiber and protein from vegetables and dal.

Cucumber Raita

Ingredients: Plain low-fat curd, diced cucumber, a pinch of roasted cumin powder, and chopped coriander.

Preparation: Mix all ingredients and chill before serving.

Nutritional Benefits: Helps with digestion and provides additional protein and fiber.

Snack 2

Chia Seed Pudding

Ingredients: Chia seeds, almond milk or low-fat milk, a few fresh berries.

Preparation: Soak chia seeds in milk overnight and top with berries before serving.

Nutritional Benefits: High in fiber, omega-3 fatty acids, and low in sugar.

Dinner

Palak (Spinach) and Paneer Curry

Ingredients: Spinach, paneer (cottage cheese), tomatoes, onions, garlic, ginger, and spices (turmeric, cumin, coriander).

Preparation: Cook spinach with spices, blend into a paste, then add paneer cubes and cook until heated through.

Nutritional Benefits: Rich in iron and protein, low in carbohydrates.

Chapati (Whole Wheat)

Ingredients: Whole wheat flour, water.

Preparation: Make the dough, roll out thinly, and cook on a griddle.

Nutritional Benefits: Whole wheat chapati has a lower glycemic index compared to refined flour.

General Tips:

<u>Portion Control</u>: Keep portions moderate to avoid excessive carbohydrate intake.

<u>Limit Added Sugars</u>: Ensure that no added sugars are included in any preparation.

<u>Include Fiber</u>: Fiber helps manage blood sugar levels effectively. Whole grains provide more fiber.

This meal plan aims to maintain stable blood sugar levels while providing balanced nutrition.

South Indian Vegetarian Meal Suggestions for Diabetic Patients.

Breakfast

1. Idli with Sambar

2. Ragi Dosa with Coconut Chutney

3. Upma with Mixed Vegetables

4. Oats Porridge with Buttermilk

5. Moong Dal Chilla (Pancake / Dosa) with Tomato Chutney

6. Puttu with Chickpeas curry. (*Puttu* is a traditional item in Kerala State, India)

Lunch

1. Brown Rice with Sambar and Vegetable Curry

2. Quinoa Biryani with Cucumber Raita

3. Millet Khichdi with Mixed Vegetable Curry

4. Red Rice with Dal and Stir-Fried Greens

5. Chapati with Sprouted Moong Dal and Cabbage Poriyal (Stir fried vegetable dish)

Dinner

1. Vegetable Pulao with Mint Raita

2. Stuffed Paratha with Low-Fat Yogurt

3. Broken Wheat Upma with Spinach Dal

4. Barley Pongal with Tomato Gotsu (Spicy Curry dish)

5. Whole Wheat Chapati with Baingan Bharta (Spicy Mashed Zucchini dish) and Curd

Snacks

1. Roasted Chana

2. Vegetable Salad with Sprouts

3. Buttermilk with Cucumber Slices

4. Mixed Nuts and Seeds

5. Fruit Salad with Low-Glycemic Fruits (e.g., Apple, Pear, Guava)

ALCOHOL AND DIABETES

Alcohol can interact with medications for diabetes, affecting blood sugar levels. Therefore, diabetics should be cautious when drinking alcohol. Also, alcohol can worsen some diabetes complications. Let us briefly explore some effects of alcohol on diabetic patients.

- Alcohol can lower blood sugar when taken with medicines like sulfonylureas and meglitinides. It also makes the pancreas produce more insulin, leading to a risk of low blood sugar. Severe low blood sugar, lasting up to 12 hours, may result from drinking alcohol. This condition is known as "*Insulin Shock*."

- Drinking alcohol on an empty stomach causes it to be absorbed quickly, increasing its effect on blood sugar. Thus, it should never be consumed without food. Always drink alcohol with a meal or snacks.
- Before drinking alcohol, like at a party, it is wise to check your blood sugar. If it is low, eat snacks or a meal before drinking alcohol.
- Since alcohol can cause dizziness and disorientation, it should be consumed slowly. Symptoms of drunkenness might actually be low blood sugar, which can be mistaken and lead to trouble with authorities like the police.
- Know your alcohol limit and how much is safe for you, as the ability to tolerate alcohol varies from person to person. If you have diabetic complications, it is best to avoid alcohol altogether.
- The American Heart Association recommends no more than two drinks per day for men and one drink per day for women who choose to drink alcohol. One drink is equivalent to:

    - 12-ounce beer (5% alcohol)

    - 8-ounce malt liquor (7% alcohol)

    - 5-ounce glass of wine (12% alcohol)

    - 1.5 ounces of 80-proof liquor

Some healthy drinks for diabetics.

Some of the healthy drinks which a diabetic may have are Seltzer water (plain unsweetened soda), Unsweetened tea or coffee, Herbal tea, Vegetable juice, Low fat or fat free milk, Buttermilk, Milk alternatives like Soy milk, Almond milk, Oat milk and Rice milk, Cashew milk, green smoothies, Sugar free lemonade, Juice of tomato, cucumber or celery.

 The Calorie content of some common beverages is given below. **(Table 1)**

Beverage	Volume (oz)	Calories
Water	8 oz	0
Coffee -unsweetened	8	2
Tea – unsweetened	8	0 -2
Whole milk	8	150
Milk 2%	8	130
Milk 1%	8	110
Milk Fat free	8	100
Fruit Juice -no sugar	8	100 - 150
Regular soda	16	130 - 250
Beer – light	12	100 - 145
Wine	5	12 - 130
Liquor 80 proof (gin, rum, whisky, vodka)	1.5 oz	95 -110

Table 1 (*See Reference: Book Ref no 1)*

Chapter 19 - MYTHS AND MISCONCEPTIONS ABOUT DIABETES

There are many myths and misconceptions about diabetes that can mislead patients and their caregivers. Some common myths include the idea that diabetes is not serious, that only overweight people get diabetes, or that eating too much sugar causes diabetes. These misconceptions can be harmful and prevent people from seeking proper treatment. It is important to get accurate information from reliable sources and healthcare professionals. Do not rely on hearsay from well-meaning but misinformed friends or family members. Always consult your doctor for the right advice. Educating yourself about diabetes will help you manage the condition better and avoid unnecessary complications. Below are some common myths regarding the condition.

This chapter further gives you some details about resources and organizations where you can get facts about the disease. It also gives you details about educational materials available from various sources.

COMMON MYTHS DEBUNKED

Myth 1: Diabetes is caused by eating too much sugar.

Reality: It is a common misconception that eating too much sugar is the sole cause of diabetes. While consuming large amounts of sugar can contribute to weight gain, which is a risk factor for developing type 2 diabetes, it is not the only cause. Diabetes is actually a complex condition influenced by various factors, including genetics and lifestyle. Type 1 diabetes, which is an autoimmune disorder, is not connected to sugar intake at all.

Explanation: To understand this better, it is important to know the difference between type 1 and type 2 diabetes. T1DM happens when the body's immune system attacks insulin-producing cells in the pancreas, and it has no link to sugar consumption. T2DM, on the other hand, involves insulin resistance and is often associated with lifestyle factors like poor diet and lack of exercise. However, genetics also plays a significant role in both types.

Myth 2: Only overweight and obese people get diabetes.

Reality: Many people believe that diabetes affects only those who are overweight or obese. While being overweight does increase the risk of developing T2DM, it is not the only factor. Diabetes can also occur in individuals who are of normal weight. T1DM, for instance, is unrelated to body weight and can develop in people of any size.

Explanation: Diabetes risk is influenced by various factors including genetics, family history, age, ethnicity, and overall medical history. For instance, someone with a family history of diabetes might be at higher risk, regardless of their weight. It is crucial to consider all these factors when understanding the risk for diabetes.

Myth 3: People with diabetes cannot eat sweets or carbohydrates.

Reality: Another common myth is that individuals with diabetes must completely avoid sweets and carbohydrates. In reality, people with diabetes can enjoy these foods in moderation as part of a balanced diet. The key is to manage portion sizes and monitor blood glucose levels carefully.

Explanation: Carbohydrate counting and understanding the glycemic index are important strategies for incorporating sweets into a diabetes-friendly diet. Carbohydrate counting involves keeping track of the amount of carbohydrates one eats, while the glycemic index measures how quickly a food raises blood sugar levels. By using these methods, people with diabetes can enjoy a variety of foods while keeping their blood sugar in check. It is always better to eat sweets along with one's meal.

Myth 4: Insulin is a cure for diabetes

Reality: Some people think that insulin is a cure for diabetes, but that is not the case. Insulin is only a treatment that helps manage blood glucose levels, but it does not *cure* the condition. Managing diabetes involves more than just taking insulin; it requires ongoing medication, a balanced diet, and lifestyle changes.

Explanation: Diabetes management is a continuous process. Even with insulin therapy, individuals with diabetes must regularly monitor their blood glucose levels and make adjustments to their treatment plan as needed. Insulin helps control blood sugar levels, but it does not eliminate the need for comprehensive diabetes management.

Myth 5: Type 2 diabetes is a mild form of diabetes

Reality: There is a misconception that T2DM is a less severe form of the disease compared to T1DM. However, this is not true. Both type 1 and type 2 diabetes are serious conditions that need careful management. Both types can lead to significant health complications which can be life threatening if not managed properly.

Explanation: T2DM can result in serious complications such as cardiovascular disease, nerve damage (*Neuropathy*), and kidney damage (*Nephropathy*). Proper management is crucial to prevent these complications and maintain overall health. It is important to recognize that both types of diabetes require diligent care and management.

Myth 6: People with diabetes cannot lead normal lives

Reality: Many people mistakenly believe that having diabetes means you cannot live a normal life. This is far from the truth. With proper management and modern treatments, people with diabetes can lead full, healthy lives.

Explanation: Advances in diabetes treatment and technology have significantly improved the quality of life for individuals with this condition. There are numerous success stories of people with diabetes who have achieved their personal and professional goals, demonstrating that diabetes does not have to limit one's life.

Myth 7: Natural or herbal remedies can cure diabetes

Reality: Some people believe that natural or herbal remedies can cure diabetes and are safer than modern medications. However, no such remedies have been proven to cure diabetes. The most effective way to manage diabetes is through established medical treatments and lifestyle changes.

Explanation: It is important to rely on evidence-based treatments for diabetes management. While some natural remedies might offer benefits, they should not replace proven medical treatments. Contrary to this, some herbal remedies may cause harm especially to the liver and the kidneys. Consulting healthcare professionals and following their recommendations is the best approach to managing diabetes.

Myth 8: Diabetes is contagious

Reality: A common misconception is that diabetes is contagious, like a cold or flu. In reality, diabetes is not contagious. It is a metabolic disorder influenced by a combination of genetic and lifestyle factors.

Explanation: Diabetes develops due to a mix of genetic predisposition and lifestyle choices. Unlike contagious diseases, it cannot be spread from person to person. Understanding how diabetes develops helps clarify that it is not something you can catch from others.

Myth 9: You cannot exercise if you have diabetes

Reality: There is a belief that people with diabetes should avoid exercise, but this is not true. In fact, regular physical activity is highly beneficial for managing diabetes. Exercise helps control blood glucose levels, improve cardiovascular health, and maintain a healthy weight.

Explanation: Engaging in regular exercise is a crucial part of diabetes management. It can help reduce blood sugar levels, enhance insulin sensitivity, and improve overall health. With proper planning and precautions, exercise is safe and advantageous for people with diabetes.

Myth 10: People with diabetes cannot donate blood

Reality: Some people believe that having diabetes disqualifies an individual from donating blood. However, those with diabetes can donate blood as long as their blood glucose levels are well-managed, and they meet other eligibility criteria for blood donation.

Explanation: Blood donation guidelines generally focus on the health and stability of the donor. If the diabetes is under control and one meets the standard health requirements, he can contribute to blood donation efforts. It is important to check with local blood donation centers for specific guidelines.

Thus, a comprehensive overview of common myths about diabetes and the factual information debunks these misconceptions. By understanding the realities behind these myths, individuals can gain a clearer and more accurate perspective on diabetes.

MORE INFORMATION AND RESOURCES

Accurate Information and Resources can be obtained from reliable sources. One should endeavor to read and understand about the disease from these sources and update one's knowledge of the disease instead of relying on information obtained from unreliable sources. Some such sources in the United States are given below.

American Diabetes Association (ADA)

The American Diabetes Association (**ADA**) is a valuable resource for anyone seeking information about diabetes. It provides a wide range of educational materials to help people understand the disease better. They also advocate for policies that improve the lives of people with diabetes and offer community programs to support those affected. By exploring their resources, individuals can access helpful guides, research updates, and support options tailored to various needs.

Centers for Disease Control and Prevention (CDC)

The Centers for Disease Control and Prevention (**CDC**) plays a crucial role in offering public health information, including data and research on diabetes and many other diseases. They provide comprehensive statistics, research findings, and educational content on how to prevent and manage diabetes. The CDC's website is an excellent source for current information and guidelines related to diabetes and other health issues.

World Health Organization (WHO)

The World Health Organization (**WHO**) provides a global perspective on diabetes management and prevention. They offer valuable insights into how diabetes is addressed worldwide, including strategies for prevention and treatment in different regions. The WHO's resources help in understanding the global efforts to combat diabetes and the various approaches taken to manage and prevent the disease.

Educational Materials

Books and Publications

There are numerous books written by healthcare professionals and diabetes experts that offer accurate and practical information. These publications provide in-depth knowledge about diabetes, including its causes, management, and treatment options. Reading these books can help individuals gain a better understanding of the condition and how to effectively manage it.

Websites and Online Platforms

Reputable websites are a great way to find up-to-date information on diabetes. Websites such as those run by the *American Diabetes Association*, the *Centers for Disease Control and Prevention*, and the *Mayo Clinic* offer valuable content on various aspects of diabetes. These online platforms provide easy access to educational resources, tips for managing diabetes, and the latest research findings.

Apps and Tools

Mobile apps and digital tools can be incredibly useful for managing diabetes. There are apps designed to help with blood glucose monitoring, meal planning, and exercise tracking. These tools can make it easier for individuals to stay on top of their diabetes management and make informed decisions about their health.

Support Networks

Diabetes Support Groups

Joining support groups can provide significant benefits for individuals with diabetes. These groups, whether local or online, offer emotional support, practical advice, and the opportunity to share experiences with others facing similar challenges. Being part of a support network can help individuals feel less isolated and more empowered in managing their condition.

Healthcare Providers

Regular consultations with healthcare providers are essential for effective diabetes management. Endocrinologists, diabetes educators, and dietitians play important roles in helping individuals understand their condition and develop a personalized management plan. Regular check-ups and professional guidance are key to maintaining good health and managing diabetes effectively.

Community Programs

Community-based programs are another valuable resource for people with diabetes. These programs offer education, resources, and support tailored to local needs. They may include workshops, health screenings, and other initiatives designed to help individuals manage their diabetes and improve their overall well-being.

Government and Non-Profit Organizations

<u>National Institutes of Health (NIH)</u>

The National Institutes of Health (**NIH**) is a major player in funding diabetes research and providing health information. The NIH supports studies that aim to advance our understanding of diabetes and improve treatment options. Their resources include research findings and information on ongoing studies that contribute to the fight against diabetes.

<u>Juvenile Diabetes Research Foundation (**JDRF**)</u>

The Juvenile Diabetes Research Foundation (JDRF) focuses on research and advocacy specifically for T1DM. They work to advance research efforts and improve the lives of individuals with T1DM through various programs and initiatives. The JDRF's work is crucial in driving forward new treatments and potential cures for type 1 diabetes.

<u>Local Health Departments</u>

Local health departments offer various resources and programs to support diabetes management and prevention within communities. These departments may provide educational materials, health screenings, and other services aimed at helping individuals manage their diabetes and prevent new cases. They are a valuable local resource for diabetes-related support. [See also next chapter on *Resources and Support*].

Educational Campaigns and Initiatives

<u>National Diabetes Prevention Program (DPP)</u>

The National Diabetes Prevention Program (**DPP**) is focused on preventing T2DM through lifestyle changes. The program emphasizes the importance of making healthy choices, such as improving diet and increasing physical activity, to reduce the risk of developing T2DM. It offers strategies and support to help people make these changes and lower their risk.

<u>Diabetes Awareness Month</u>

Diabetes Awareness Month is an important time for raising awareness about diabetes and promoting early detection and effective management. During this month, various activities and campaigns are organized to educate the public about diabetes, its risks, and the importance of early intervention. Participating in these events can help spread knowledge and support efforts to combat diabetes.

These explanations aim to provide comprehensive guidance on debunking common myths and offering accurate information and resources for readers. By exploring these resources and understanding the facts, individuals can better manage their diabetes and support others in their journey.

Sources of Educational Materials in India

There are some sources of educational materials, support groups, and associations in India that offer valuable information and support for diabetes management and education. Some of these are given below.

Diabetes Foundation India (DFI)

Website:[Diabetes Foundation of India]
https://www.diabetesfoundationindia.org/

DFI provides a wealth of information on diabetes management, including educational materials, research updates, and guidelines. They offer resources for patients, healthcare professionals, and the general public.

Indian Diabetes Association (IDA)

IDA focuses on diabetes education and awareness through various programs and publications. They offer resources such as brochures, booklets, and information on diabetes care.

National Diabetes, Obesity and Cholesterol Foundation (N-DOC)

https://www.facebook.com/NdocFoundation/

N-DOC provides educational materials, guidelines, and resources for diabetes management. They focus on patient education and offer workshops and seminars on diabetes and related conditions.

All India Institute of Medical Sciences (AIIMS)

Website: [AIIMS Delhi] (https://www.aiims.edu/)

AIIMS Delhi, one of India's premier medical institutions, offers educational resources and research on diabetes. Their website includes information on diabetes care and research findings.

Mayo Clinic India

Website: [Mayo Clinic India] (https://www.mayoclinic.org/)

Mayo Clinic India offers comprehensive resources on diabetes management, including educational articles and guidelines. They provide expert advice and practical information for patients.

Support Groups and Associations

Diabetes India

Website : [Diabetes India] (https://www.diabetesindia.com/)

Diabetes India is a leading organization dedicated to diabetes education and support. They provide resources, patient support groups, and information on diabetes management. They also organize events and workshops for public awareness.

The Diabetic Association of India (DAI)

DAI is a prominent organization that offers support for diabetes patients through education, advocacy, and community programs. They provide information on diabetes care and manage various support groups across India.

Indian Association of Diabetes Educators (IADE)

IADE focuses on diabetes education and professional development. They offer resources for both patients and healthcare professionals, including educational workshops and certification programs.

Diabetes Self-Management Education (DSME) India

DSME India provides education and support for diabetes management. They offer workshops, online resources, and support groups to help individuals manage their diabetes effectively.

Local Health Departments and Hospitals

Many local health departments and hospitals across India offer diabetes education and support programs. Check with local hospitals and clinics for resources and support groups in your area.

Educational Campaigns and Initiatives

National Diabetes Awareness Campaigns

Various national and regional campaigns focus on raising awareness about diabetes and promoting education. Look for campaigns organized by diabetes associations, healthcare providers, and government health departments.

World Diabetes Day Events

Celebrated on November 14th each year, World Diabetes Day features events and activities aimed at increasing diabetes awareness and education. Many organizations in India participate in these events to provide information and support.

These resources should provide comprehensive support for diabetes education and management in India. [See also chapter 20 on *Resources and Support*].

Chapter 20 - RESOURCES AND SUPPORT

Managing diabetes effectively requires access to reliable resources and a strong support network. In this chapter, we will explore various avenues where patients can find information and assistance. Trusted sources such as healthcare providers, diabetes educators, and registered dietitians offer personalized guidance on managing diabetes, including medication, diet, and lifestyle adjustments. Online platforms and organizations, like the American Diabetes Association and the International Diabetes Federation, provide a wealth of information, from educational materials to the latest research updates. Support groups, both in-person and online, can offer emotional support and practical advice from others who understand the daily challenges of living with diabetes. By utilizing these resources and support systems, patients can make informed decisions, stay motivated, and improve their overall well-being.

The details regarding many of these organizations and associations in the United States and India have already been discussed before in the previous chapter. Some of the resources in the United Kingdom are discussed below.

Diabetes UK (https://www.diabetes.org.uk/)

Diabetes UK is dedicated to supporting people with diabetes in the United Kingdom. Their efforts include conducting research, advocating for better diabetes care, and providing educational resources to help people manage their diabetes. They work to improve the lives of those affected by diabetes through various programs and initiatives.

Diabetes UK is actively involved in community engagement through programs like Diabetes Week, which raises awareness about diabetes and promotes better management practices. They also organize fundraising events and offer peer support groups where individuals can connect with others facing similar challenges.

Diabetes UK offers a range of resources including educational materials and guides on managing diabetes. They provide helplines for support and information, and their website is a valuable resource for up-to-date information on diabetes care.

Local and Regional Organizations

Local diabetes organizations play a vital role in providing support and resources tailored to the specific needs of their communities. These organizations offer programs and services that address local concerns and provide practical help for managing diabetes.

Examples of local organizations include State Diabetes Associations, which focus on regional issues and support, Hospital-Based Diabetes Centers that offer specialized care, and Community Health Programs that provide educational workshops and health fairs. These organizations are crucial for providing accessible support and resources.

Local and regional organizations typically offer a variety of resources such as educational workshops, health fairs, and support groups. These resources help individuals manage their diabetes more effectively and connect with others in their community who are facing similar challenges.

A detailed overview of organizations and associations should help readers find valuable resources and support for managing diabetes.

Online Communities and Forums

<u>Peer Support</u>: Online communities and forums are valuable resources for connecting with other people who have similar experiences with diabetes. These platforms provide a space where you can share your own experiences, ask questions, and receive support from others who understand what you are going through. Engaging with these communities can offer emotional support and practical advice from people who have firsthand experience with diabetes.

<u>Popular Platforms</u>: There are several popular online forums and communities where you can find support and information about diabetes. *TuDiabetes* is a well-known community where members share their experiences and advice on managing diabetes. *Diabetes Daily* is another popular forum that provides a space for discussion and support. Reddit also has a dedicated forum, *r/diabetes*, where users share their stories and offer tips on living with diabetes.

<u>Benefits</u>: Joining online communities has numerous benefits. You can gain emotional support from others who understand the challenges of living with diabetes. These forums also offer practical advice on managing the condition, including tips for dealing with specific symptoms or situations. Sharing personal experiences can help you feel less isolated and more connected to others who face similar challenges.

Social Media Groups

Platforms: Social media platforms are another great way to connect with others and find information about diabetes. Facebook, Twitter, and Instagram all host groups and pages dedicated to diabetes where you can follow updates and engage with content related to diabetes care and support. *But be careful not to share your personal data on these platforms*.

Engagement: These social media groups facilitate engagement through discussions, question-and-answer sessions, and the sharing of tips and personal stories. You can participate in conversations, ask questions about managing diabetes, and learn from the experiences of others. These interactions can help you stay informed and find support from a broad community.

Examples of popular social media groups include Facebook groups focused on diabetes support, such as those for type 1 or type 2 diabetes. On Twitter (X), hashtags like *#DiabetesCommunity*, *#Type1Diabetes*, and *#Type2Diabetes* can lead you to useful discussions and resources. Instagram also features hashtags and pages where individuals and organizations share insights, tips, and personal stories about living with diabetes. *Be discrete and careful while exchanging information on these social media platforms.*

Mobile Apps

Diabetes Management Apps: Mobile apps play a significant role in helping people manage their diabetes by providing tools to track various aspects of their health. These apps can help you monitor your blood glucose levels, track your diet, and log your exercise routines. By using these apps, you can keep detailed records of your health and make more informed decisions about your diabetes management.

Popular Apps: There are several popular apps designed for diabetes management. For example, *MySugr* is an app that helps you log your blood glucose levels and provides insights into your trends. *Glucose Buddy* is another app that offers features for tracking your glucose levels, medication, and meals. *One Drop* is an app that integrates with other health devices and provides personalized recommendations based on your data.

When choosing a diabetes management app, look for features that will be most useful to you. Key features to consider include data logging, which allows you to keep track of your glucose levels and other health metrics. Trend analysis helps you understand patterns in your data, and reminders can assist you in taking your medications or checking your blood glucose levels at the right times. Integration with other health devices can also be beneficial for a more comprehensive approach to managing your diabetes.

This description provides a thorough overview of online resources and communities available for diabetes education and support which the patient can access from anywhere.

Books and Publications

Educational Books

Comprehensive Guides: If one is looking for in-depth and easy-to-understand information about diabetes, there are several excellent comprehensive guides available. For example, *"Diabetes for Dummies"* by Dr. Alan L. Rubin is a great choice. This book provides a thorough overview of diabetes in simple language. Another excellent guide is *"Think Like a Pancreas"* by Gary Scheiner. This book offers practical advice and strategies for managing diabetes, making it easier for you to understand and apply the information in your daily life. *"Mayo Clinic the Essential Diabetes book"* by M. Regina Castro is another very useful book.

Specific Topics: For those interested in specific aspects of diabetes management, there are books that focus on particular topics. "*Bright Spots & Landmines*" by Adam Brown is a fantastic resource for practical tips on managing diabetes effectively. It provides actionable advice and strategies that can help you navigate the challenges of living with diabetes.

Research-Based Books: If one is interested in research-based information, "*Dr. Bernstein's Diabetes Solution*" by Dr. Richard K. Bernstein is a notable choice. This book presents a detailed approach to diabetes management based on extensive research and clinical experience, offering insights into controlling blood sugar levels and improving overall health.

Cookbooks and Nutrition Guides

Healthy Recipes: When it comes to managing diabetes, having access to healthy and delicious recipes is essential. Cookbooks like "*The Diabetes Cookbook*" by the American Diabetes Association are excellent resources. This book includes a variety of recipes specifically designed to help manage diabetes while still enjoying flavorful meals. Another great option is "*The Complete Diabetes Cookbook*" by America's Test Kitchen. This cookbook provides a wide range of recipes that are both nutritious and easy to prepare.

Meal Planning: For those looking to plan their meals and follow nutritional guidelines, books like "*The Diabetes Plate Method*" by the American Diabetes Association are highly recommended. This book focuses on practical meal planning strategies and offers guidance on how to create balanced meals that support diabetes management.

Special Diets: If you have specific dietary preferences, there are cookbooks tailored to different diets. For example, "*The Mediterranean Diabetes Cookbook*" by Amy Riolo offers recipes that follow the Mediterranean diet, which is known for its health benefits and can be particularly helpful for managing diabetes.

Some books published in India

This is a list of a few notable cookbooks and nutrition guides for diabetics published in India.

"The Complete Diabetes Cookbook" by America's Test Kitchen. This book offers over 400 diabetes-friendly recipes that emphasize both flavor and nutrition. Each recipe is vetted by a dietitian and a doctor, ensuring it meets specific nutritional guidelines. It is a comprehensive resource for anyone looking to manage diabetes through healthy eating.

"Low GI Diet Managing Type 2 Diabetes" This guide provides clear and simple advice on what to eat and do to manage T2DM effectively. It includes practical tips on choosing the best carbohydrates and managing your diet to reduce diabetes-related complications.

"CSIRO Low-Carb Diabetes Diet & Lifestyle Solution" is a book featuring 80 recipes and twelve weeks of meal plans. This book offers a lifestyle solution that can help with weight loss and improving metabolic health and blood glucose control.

There are also many more such books published in India by chefs and individuals. These resources can be immensely helpful for anyone looking to manage diabetes through diet and lifestyle changes.

Dr. Gauri Rokkam - Author of *"Diabetic Recipes."*

Tarla Dalal - Renowned Indian cookbook author who has written *"Healthy Diabetic Recipes."*

Nita Mehta - A well-known chef and author who has penned *"Diabetic Snacks & Low Calorie Cooking."*

Sanjeev Kapoor - Famous chef with a series of cookbooks, including *"Healthy Tiffin & Snacks for Diabetics."* Also *"Healthy Indian Cooking for Diabetes"* by him.

"The Diabetic Cookbook" by Sastha Press.

"Indian Recipes for Diabetic Patients" by Tod Bruffee.

"Indian Low Carb Recipes" by Dr. Paramesh Shamanna et al.

These authors have created recipes that cater to the dietary needs of diabetics, offering a variety of dishes that help manage blood sugar levels while being tasty and satisfying for Indian tastes. Many of them are available online on **Amazon.in**.

Personal Stories and Memoirs

<u>Inspiring Journeys</u>: Reading personal stories and memoirs can provide valuable insight and inspiration. *"Breakthrough"* by Lisa Hepner is a memoir that shares an inspiring journey with diabetes, offering a personal perspective on living with the condition. *"Balancing Diabetes"* by Kerri Sparling is another memoir that provides a heartfelt account of the author's experiences with diabetes, offering encouragement and motivation to readers.

<u>Diverse Perspectives</u>: Books that share diverse experiences with diabetes can offer additional perspectives and insights. *"The Book of Better"* by Chuck Eichten is a compelling read that provides practical advice through personal experiences. *"Sugar Linings: Finding the Bright Side of Type 1 Diabetes"* by Sierra Anne Sandison is another great book that shares a positive outlook on managing T1DM and finding joy despite the challenges.

Magazines and Journals

<u>Monthly Magazines</u>: For ongoing updates, tips, and stories related to diabetes, consider subscribing to diabetes-specific magazines. *Diabetes Forecast* (published by the American Diabetes Association) and *Diabetic Living* are both excellent choices. These magazines offer a variety of articles on diabetes management, recipes, and personal stories that can keep you informed and engaged.

<u>Academic Journals</u>: If one is interested in the latest research and scientific studies, academic journals are a valuable resource. Journals like *Diabetes Care*, *Diabetes*, and *The Lancet Diabetes & Endocrinology* publish cutting-edge research and clinical studies related to diabetes, providing insights into new treatments and findings in the field.

<u>Newsletter Subscriptions</u>: Subscribing to newsletters from organizations like the American Diabetes Association (ADA), the Juvenile Diabetes Research Foundation (JDRF), and the International Diabetes Federation (IDF) is another way to stay informed. These newsletters offer regular updates, research highlights, and practical tips for managing diabetes. These are helpful for patients as well as caregivers of diabetic patients.

By exploring these books and publications, a person can gain a wealth of knowledge and support to help navigate the diabetes journey with confidence. Each resource offers valuable information and insights that can assist the diabetic in managing the condition effectively.

REFERENCES

BOOKS

1. Davidson's Principles and Practice of Medicine. Edited by Ralston SH, Penman, ID Strachan MWJ, Hobson RP. 23rd Edition. 2018. Elsevier Ltd.
2. Diabetes for Dummies. Dr. Simon Poole, Amy Riolo. Alan L Rubin. 6th Edition, 2023. John Wiley & Sons.
3. Mayo Clinic. The Essential Diabetes Book. M Regina Castro. 2022. Mayo Clinic Press.
4. Diabetes and the Cardiovascular System. McGuire DK. In Braunwald's Heart Disease. Vol II. Edited by Mann DL, Zipes DP, Libby P, Bonow RO. 10th Edition. 2015

REFERENCES

1. Type 2 Diabetes mellitus: A Review of Current Trends. Oman Med J. Jul; 27(4): 269–273. 2022.
2. Standards of Care in Diabetes. 2024. Diabetes Care. Vol 47. Supplemnt. 1, Jan 2024.
3. History of Diabetes. Wikipedia. 2024.
4. Milestones in the History of Diabetes mellitus. Karamanou M, Protogerou A, et al. World J Diabetes. Jan 10; 7(1): 1–7. 2016.
5. Type 1 Diabetes. Medline plus 2024.

6. About Type 1 Diabetes. Center for Disease Control. May 15, 2024.

7. Epidemiology, presentation, and diagnosis of type 2 diabetes mellitus in children and adolescents. Laffel L, Svoren B. Up To Date. 2023.

8. Management of type 2 diabetes mellitus in children and adolescents. Laffel L, Svoren B. Up To Date. 2023.

9. Type 1 Diabetes. StatPearls [Internet]. National Library of Medicine. Jessica Lucier; Ruth S. Weinstock. 2023.

10. Current Advances in the Management of Diabetes Mellitus. Aloke C, Egwu CO, Aja PM. Biomedicines. Oct; 10(10): 2436. 2022.

11. Patient education: Type 2 diabetes and diet (Beyond the Basics). Delahanty LM. Up To Date. 2024.

12. Medical nutrition therapy for type 2 diabetes mellitus. Up To Date 2024.

13. Chronic complications and screening in children and adolescents with type 2 diabetes mellitus. Up To Date. 2023.

14. : Overview of the musculoskeletal complications of diabetes mellitus. Up To Date. 2023.

15. Healthy diet in adults. Up To Date. 2023.

16. Glycemic management and vascular complications in type 2 diabetes mellitus. Up To Date. 2023.

17. Overview of general medical care in nonpregnant adults with diabetes mellitus. Up To Date. 2023.

18. Diabetes mellitus in the elderly. Chentli.F, AzzougS, Mahgoun.S, Indian J of Endocrinology & Metabolism. 2015, 19: 744-752.

19. Exercice & type 2 diabetes. Colberg SR et al. Diabetes Care. 2010. Dec. 33: 147-167

20. Internet Interventions to Support Lifestyle Modification for Diabetes Management: A Systematic Review of the Evidence. Cotterez A, Durant N et al.   J Diabetes Complications. 28 (2): 243-251. 2015.

21. Indian Vegetarian Diet Chart for Diabetic Patients. Felix Hospitals. 2024.

22. 45 Food Items that may Help Control Blood Sugar. Kukude I. PharmEasy. 2024.

23. What An Ideal Indian Diabetes-friendly Diet Plan Looks Like. Anvayaa. Feb. 2021.

24. National Diabetes Statistical Report 2024. Center for Diseases Control.

25. Diabetic Perioperative Management. Dogra P; Anastasopoulou C; Jialal I. Stat Pearls [Internet] National Library of Medicine. Jan 2024.

26. Statistics about Diabetes: American Diabetes Association. 2021.

27. Divers J, Mayer-Davis EJ, Lawrence JM, et al. Trends in Incidence of Type 1 and Type 2 Diabetes Among Youths — Selected Counties and Indian Reservations, United States, 2002–2015. MMWR Morb Mortal Wkly Rep 2020;69:161–165.

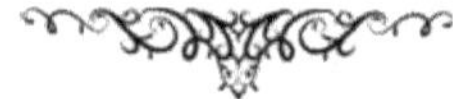

APPENDIX

<u>Conversion Tables Weights And Measures</u>

Weights

1 lb. = 0.45 kg   1 kg = 2.2 lbs.   1 oz (weight) = 28 g

Volumes

1 US cup = 237 milliliters (mL)

1 teaspoon = 5 milliliters (ml)

1 tablespoon = 15 milliliters (ml)

1 ounce (volume) = 30 milliliters. (ml)

Temperature conversion

Celsius to Fahrenheit $°F = (°C × 9/5) + 32$

Fahrenheit to Celsius $°C = (°F - 32) × 5/9$

For converting Lipids (cholesterol, LDL, HDL and Non-HDL Cholesterol)

1 mg/dL of cholesterol   =   0.025 mmol/L

1 mmol/L = 38.7 mg/L

For converting Triglycerides

mg/dl   to mmol/L   1 mg/dL = 0.01 mmol/L

mmol/L to mg/dL   1 mmol/L = 89 mg/dL

To convert from mg/dL to mmol/L, you divide the mg/dL value by 89 (the molecular weight of triglycerides in g/mol).

To convert from mmol/L to mg/dL, you multiply the mmol/L value by 89.

For converting Glucose

1 mmol/L = 18 mg/dL

1 mg/dL = 0.06 mmol/L

ACKNOWLEDGEMENT

I owe immense gratitude to my family for their unwavering support throughout the process of writing this book. Their encouragement has been invaluable. My daughter, Sandya, has been especially helpful, guiding me through the nuances of computer use and assisting with the text formatting and preparation of the QR codes for my books.

My sincere gratitude goes to Prof. R. Krishnan, Senior Physician at Baby Memorial Hospital, Calicut, who generously provided me with invaluable references and resources essential for the creation of this book.

I am also deeply thankful to my colleagues in the author community, who generously assisted me and provided constructive feedback on my previous works. They have been quick to offer advice whenever I faced challenges in my writing.

Special recognition goes to Mr. Som Bathla, my mentor on this journey, and to the members of the Author-Helping-Author (AHA) community, whose guidance has been instrumental in shaping my writing and publishing endeavors.

My teachers in the medical schools where I received my undergraduate and postgraduate training deserve special mention. I have achieved what I have by standing on the shoulders of these stalwarts who taught me the art and science of medicine. My deepest respect and gratitude go to them.

MORE BOOKS BY THE AUTHOR

<u>NON-FICTION</u>

How to Face the Challenges while Growing Old Problems
of Elderly Book 1

Old Age Health Challenges and Solutions Problems
of Elderly Book 2

Understanding the Electrocardiogram Medical
Book on ECG

Demystifying Hinduism
Understanding Hinduism Book 1

The Avadhoota – Whispers of Wisdom
Understanding Hinduism Book 2

Daily Musings
Understanding Hinduism Book 3

How to Master Essential Life Skills Skill sets for
Success Book 1

How to Achieve Professional Excellence Skill sets for
Success Book 2

<u>FICTION</u>

Tell Me a Story, Grandpa Short Stories for Children
Book 1

Grandpa, Tell me More Stories Short Stories for Children
Book 2

In Search of a Bridegroom An Autobiographical Fiction

The Truth Lies Out There A Family Drama of Suspense

Code Black A Hospital based Thriller

About the Author

Dr. K. V. Sahasranam MD, DM, FACC, FCSI, is a distinguished Cardiologist and former Professor of Cardiology at Calicut Medical College, India. With over 45 years of medical practice, he has retired and now resides in the USA. His deep passion lies in educating students and residents, reflected in his book, "**Understanding the Electrocardiogram**," designed for medical students and physicians, which thoroughly explores the ECG and simplifies its interpretation. Additionally, Dr. Sahasranam offers a comprehensive *3-module course on ECG* through the Udemy platform.

Writing under the pen name *'Sahasranam Kalpathy,'* he has authored 12 more books, spanning both fiction and nonfiction. His works include a series on *'Problems of the Elderly'* (2 books), *'Understanding Hinduism'* (3 books), *'Skillsets for Success'* (2 books), three captivating Fiction novels and two books of Short stories for children. All of his books are available on **Amazon** and **Notionpress.com** (India).

This latest book is the first part of the *'Everyday Health Guide'* series.

WEBSITE: **kvsauthor.com**